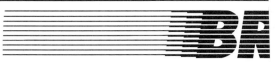 

EASY 4-STEP
METHOD TO
DRUG CALCULATIONS

S. D. FOUST

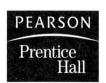

Upper Saddle River, New Jersey

Library of Congress Cataloging-in-Publication Data

Foust, S. D.
   Easy 4-step method to drug calculations / S. D. Foust.
      p. ; cm.
Includes bibliographical references and index.
   ISBN 0-13-113460-4 (pbk.)
   1. Pharmaceutical arithmetic. 2. Solutions (Pharmacy)
[DNLM: 1. Pharmaceutical Preparations—administration & dosage—Programmed Instruction. 2. Mathematics—
Programmed Instruction. QV 18.2 F782e 2004] I. Title: Easy four step method to drug calculations. II. Title.

RS57.F68 2004
615′. 14—dc22

2003026341

Publisher: Julie Levin Alexander
Publisher's Assistant: Regina Bruno
Senior Acquisitions Editor: Tiffany Price Salter
Editorial Assistant: Joanna Rodzen-Hickey
Senior Marketing Manager: Katrin Beacom
Channel Marketing Manager: Rachele Strober
Director of Production and Manufacturing: Bruce Johnson
Managing Editor for Production: Patrick Walsh
Production Liaison: Julie Li
Production Editor: Karen Ettinger, *The GTS Companies*/York, PA Campus
Manufacturing Manager: Ilene Sanford
Manufacturing Buyer: Pat Brown
Creative Director: Cheryl Asherman
Senior Design Coordinator: Christopher Weigand
Cover Designer: Christopher Weigand
Cover Image: Don Bishop/Getty Images, Inc.
Composition: *The GTS Companies*/York, PA Campus
Printing and Binding: The Banta Company
Cover Printer: Coral Graphics

Pearson Education Ltd.
Pearson Education Singapore Pte. Ltd.
Pearson Education Canada, Ltd.
Pearson Education—Japan

Pearson Education Australia Pty. Limited
Pearson Education North Asia Ltd.
Pearson Educación de Mexico, S.A. de C.V.
Pearson Education Malaysia Pte. Ltd.

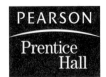

10 9 8 7 6 5 4 3 2 1
ISBN 0-13-113460-4

Dedication

This instructional guide is dedicated to the thousands of health care providers, in both the emergency and clinical fields, who have administered lifesaving measures to the millions of sick and injured patients treated every year. The pre-hospital emergency personnel, nurses, physicians, and other health care providers are to be commended for a job well done, without reservation. This book will assist in the development of many more outstanding professionals.

Preface

Easy 4-Step Method To Drug Calculations was first self published by the author in 1993 and distributed throughout various facilities and colleges in the United States and abroad. In 1996, this manual was revised, updated, and self published as a second edition. After developing a reputation for its simplicity and demand in both classroom environments and field application, it has been professionally designed, updated, and published. This material will now be able to reach a much broader span of its intended audience, and will most assuredly be a powerful tool in the development of many great health care providers.

This book is your guide to calculating liquid drug administrations via **subcutaneous, intramuscular, intravenous push, intravenous drip, endotracheal,** or **intraosseous infusion.** The text identifies, in detail, the simplest form of a 4-step method that can be used on any of the previously mentioned routes. Please refer to it when you need instruction or review, or when you have any question about calculating liquid drug dosages.

Designed especially for **paramedics, nurses, students,** and other **health care professionals,** as well as **colleges, universities,** and other **advanced training facilities,** this book is written with the intention of clearly explaining every step. It addresses complications that one may encounter while calculating drug dosages. It is designed to eliminate confusion and increase awareness during each calculation.

In an effort to maintain simplicity and practicality, we have tried to use doses and concentrations commonly found in use today when we cite examples and questions. Manufacturer or protocols may change the dose or concentration, but the four easy steps will still apply.

The **objective** of this book is to teach only the information necessary for learning and calculating drug dosages. Excessive information often leads to confusion and discouragement. This book is very elementary, easy to read and follow. By the time you complete the reading and learning of this material, you will feel much more confident in your understanding and capabilities in calculating drug dosages.

REFERENCES AND ACKNOWLEDGMENTS

Bledsoe, B. E., Porter, R. S., and Shade, B. R. (1994). *Paramedic Emergency Care,* 2nd ed. Prentice Hall.

Caroline, N. (1991). *Emergency Care in the Streets,* 4th ed. Little, Brown.

Grauer, K. and Cavallaro, D. (1993). *Advanced Cardiac Life Support,* 3rd ed. Mosby Lifeline.

Nurse's Drug Handbook, (1993). W. B. Saunders.

CONTRIBUTORS

A special thanks to those who gave freely of their time to contribute their ideas and suggestions. These EMS experts, coworkers, and friends are to be well commended for their assistance in the preparation of this book.

REVIEWERS

The reviewers provided excellent ideas, suggestions, and many positive comments on this book. These reviews are deeply appreciated.

Overview

The objective of this overview is to give the reader an insight or general idea of the material that will be presented. It is important to remember that in an effort to maintain simplicity and practicality, the author has tried to use doses and concentrations commonly found in use today when he cites examples and questions. Manufacturer or protocols may change the dose or concentration of a medication, but the four easy steps will still apply.

The introduction begins by teaching the abbreviations and conversions essential for properly understanding and calculating this easy 4-step formula. The following four chapters go on to teach and explain, in clear detail, the most simplified formula used in calculating drug dosages.

Each chapter will correlate in number to each step in the calculation formula. Thus, Chapter 1 will deal with step 1, Chapter 2 will deal with step 2, and so forth. In an effort to familiarize the reader with the four steps of this formula, what follows is a brief description of each.

Chapter 1 explains the process of identifying and calculating, if necessary, step 1 of the formula, which is establishing the desired dose (**DD**).

Establish the desired dose (**DD**). **DD** is defined as the amount of a particular drug to be administered. When an order has been given either verbally, by protocol, or other means, you must first be able to identify the desired dose and separate it from the other information given. At times it becomes necessary to calculate the desired dose, as explained further in the chapter.

Step 1   DD

Chapter 2 explains the process for calculating step 2 of the formula, which is calculating the concentration (**C**).

> Calculate the concentration (**C**) of the drug being administered. The concentration is the total weight of the drug (normally gm, mg, μg, and units) mixed in a total amount of cc's (ml's).
>
> | Step 1 | DD |
> |--------|----|
> | **Step 2** | **C (always weight/cc)** |
> | | **e.g.—mg/cc** |

Chapter 3 explains the process for calculating step 3 of the formula, which will result in the number of cc's to be delivered to achieve the desired dose (DD).

> Calculate the amount of cc's to be delivered. There are two reasons for this particular calculation: (1) when giving a drug through sq., IM, IV, ET, or IO, it is necessary to calculate the amount of cc's to be drawn from a particular container (ampule or vial) or to be pushed through a prefilled syringe so that the desired dose can be delivered, or (2) to calculate the amount of cc's needed to figure gtts/min, which is required in step 4, calculating drip rates. For whichever reason cc's are being calculated, the formula is:
>
> | Step 1 | DD |
> |--------|----|
> | Step 2 | C |
> | **Step 3** | $\dfrac{DD}{C}$ |

Chapter 4 explains the process for calculating step 4 of the formula, which is calculating the drip rate.

> Calculate the drip rate. Calculating the drip rate is required to deliver the desired dose. The formula is:
>
> | Step 1 | DD |
> |--------|----|
> | Step 2 | C |
> | Step 3 | $\dfrac{DD}{C}$ |
> | **Step 4** | $\dfrac{cc \times gtt}{time}$ |

Contents

Conversions

ABBREVIATIONS

Listed below are the abbreviations that will be used in this calculation guide:

C—concentration	**IO**—intraosseous	**mEq**—milliequivilant
cc—cubic centimeter	**IV**—intravenous	**mg**—milligram
DD—desired dose	**IVP**—intravenous push	**min**—minute
ET—endotracheal	**kg**—kilogram	**ml**—milliliter
gm—gram	**lb**—pound/pounds	**sq**—subcutaneous
gtt—drop/drops	**L**—liter	**μg**—microgram
IM—intramuscular	**mcg**—microgram	

Now that the abbreviations have been established, converting one measurement to another needs to be addressed. It is extremely important to **memorize** the conversion procedure to be able to promptly calculate drug dosages and drug administrations using the formula taught in this guide.

Nearly all drugs are supplied in gm, mg, and μg. If by chance you find a drug that is not found in one of the above mentioned measurements, simply **plug** it into the outlined formula. The units of measure used in this guide are gm, mg, μg, mEq, units, L, ml, and cc. This guide will teach only those conversions that are necessary to know when dealing both with this particular formula and liquid drug administration.

CONVERTING gm TO mg

When converting **gm** to **mg,** move the decimal point **three** places to the **right.** See examples:

$$1.0 \, gm = 1\underset{1\,2\,3}{0\,0\,0}. \, mg \qquad 1.5 \, gm = 1\underset{1\,2\,3}{5\,0\,0}. \, mg$$

(Note the movement of the decimal point **three** places to the **right.**)

Since mg are **smaller** than gm, the **number** in mg will be **larger** than the **number** in gm. See examples:

$$\mathbf{1000} \, mg = \mathbf{1.0} \, gm \qquad \mathbf{1500} \, mg = \mathbf{1.5} \, gm$$

As noted below, there are 1000 mg in 1.0 gm. See example:

$$\mathbf{1000} \, mg = \mathbf{1.0} \, gm$$

CONVERTING mg TO µg

When converting **mg** to **µg,** the same format is used. **Move** the decimal point **three** places to the **right.** See examples:

$$1.0 \, mg = 1\underset{1\,2\,3}{0\,0\,0}. \, \mu g \qquad 1.5 \, mg = 1\underset{1\,2\,3}{5\,0\,0}. \, \mu g$$

(Note the movement of the decimal point **three** places to the **right.**)

Since µg are **smaller** than mg, the **number** in µg will be **larger** than the **number** in mg. See examples:

$$\mathbf{1000} \, \mu g = \mathbf{1.0} \, mg \qquad \mathbf{1500} \, \mu g = \mathbf{1.5} \, mg$$

As noted below, there are 1000 µg in 1.0 mg. See example:

$$\mathbf{1000} \, \mu g = \mathbf{1.0} \, mg$$

CONVERTING L TO ml

When converting **L** to **ml,** the same format is used. **Move** the decimal point **three** places to the **right.** See examples:

$$1.0 \, L = 1\underset{1\,2\,3}{0\,0\,0}. \, ml \qquad 1.5 \, L = 1\underset{1\,2\,3}{5\,0\,0}. \, ml$$

(Note the movement of the decimal point **three** places to the **right.**)

Since ml are **smaller** than L, the **number** in ml will be **larger** than the **number** in L. See examples:

$$1000 \text{ ml} = 1.0 \text{ L} \qquad 1500 \text{ ml} = 1.5 \text{ L}$$

As noted below, there are 1000 ml in 1.0 L. See example:

$$1000 \text{ ml} = 1.0 \text{ L}$$

As you have now learned, **moving** the decimal point to the **right** means that a **larger** unit of measure has been converted to a **smaller** unit of measure (e.g. gm to mg), thus creating a **larger** number. Always remember, the **smaller** the unit of measure, the **larger** the number.

Regarding **ml's** and **cc's,** no conversion takes place between these two measurements because they are interchangeable when used in liquid drug administrations and in using this particular formula taught in this guide. See examples:

$$1 \text{ ml} = 1 \text{ cc} \qquad 1.5 \text{ ml} = 1.5 \text{ cc}$$

CONVERTING lb TO kg

Prior to calculating kg's, make note of the following points:

1. *Whole numbers* are those to the **left** of the decimal point. See examples:

$$123. \qquad 456. \qquad 789.$$

2. *Decimal fractions* are those numbers to the **right** of the decimal point. See examples:

$$.123 \qquad .456 \qquad .789$$

3. *Dividend* is the number being **divided** (the number **within** the division bar). See examples:

$$\overline{)36} \qquad \overline{)72} \qquad \overline{)144}$$

4. *Divisor* is the number used to **divide** another (the number found to the **left** of the division bar). See examples:

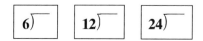

5. The *answer* (number found **above** the division bar) is the end result of the **dividend** being divided by the **divisor.** See examples:

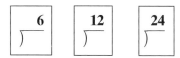

In conclusion:

$$\mathbf{Divisor} = 6\overline{)36} \begin{matrix} 6 = \mathbf{Answer} \\ = \mathbf{Dividend} \end{matrix}$$

The above example reads: **36** divided by **6** equals **6.**

Study and be familiar with all of the above definitions before continuing with the conversion of lb to kg.

When converting **lb** to **kg,** divide the **pounds** by **2.2.**

See examples:

$$2.2\overline{)220}\ \text{lb} \qquad 2.2\overline{)165}\ \text{lb}$$

Sometimes when calculating this conversion on paper, these numbers tend to get reversed in reference to the divisor being in the dividend place and the dividend being in the divisor place. **To avoid this complication,** say to yourself, for example:`

220 lb [write that down], **divided by** [draw the division bar around the $\overline{)200}$], **2.2** [write that down in the divisor place—$2.2\overline{)220}$].

In reference to the decimal in the previous example, the division process can be simplified by moving the decimal in the **divisor** (2.2) to the **right** one place, thus converting this decimal number to a **whole number.** It is much easier to divide a whole number by a whole number. See example:

$$2.2\overline{)} \qquad \longrightarrow \qquad 2\,2.\overline{)}$$

At the same time, **move** the **decimal** point in the **dividend** one place to the **right** and **insert a zero** in its place. See example:

$$\overline{)220\ 0.} \qquad \longrightarrow \qquad \overline{)2200}$$

Remember, whenever a decimal point is moved, creating a larger number, replace it with a zero. Eliminating the decimal point eliminates the concern of being sure that the point is placed in the correct spot in the answer. See examples:

$$2.2 \overline{)220} \text{ lb} \longrightarrow 2\underset{1}{2,} \overline{)220\underset{\smile}{\underline{0}}} \text{ lb} \begin{array}{r} 100\text{ kg} \\ \underline{-22} \\ 0 \end{array} \quad \text{or} \quad \frac{220}{2.2} \longrightarrow \frac{220\underline{0}}{2\underset{1}{2_{\smile}}} = 100 \text{ kg}$$

Always keep a mental note when calculating this conversion that the number in kg is slightly less than half of the number in lb. See example:

$$\boxed{\textbf{100} \text{ kg} = \textbf{220} \text{ lb}}$$

If the **answer** in kg contains **one** or **more** decimal fractions, then the answer needs to be **rounded off** to the nearest **whole number.** If the decimal fraction is **.5** or **higher,** then the **whole number** needs to be **increased by one,** eliminating all decimal fractions. See examples:

$$\boxed{20.\textbf{5} \longrightarrow 21} \quad \boxed{20.\textbf{6} \longrightarrow 21} \quad \boxed{20.\textbf{9} \longrightarrow 21}$$

If the decimal fraction is **.4** or **less,** the whole number will **remain** the same, at the same time completely eliminating the decimal fractions in the answer. See examples:

$$\boxed{20.\textbf{4} \longrightarrow 20} \quad \boxed{20.\textbf{3} \longrightarrow 20} \quad \boxed{20.\textbf{1} \longrightarrow 20}$$

Again, each decimal fraction needs to be rounded off until they are all eliminated. See examples:

$$
\begin{array}{ll}
20.\textbf{7} \longrightarrow \textbf{21} & 34.\textbf{42} \longrightarrow 34.\textbf{4} \longrightarrow \textbf{34} \\
54.\textbf{8} \longrightarrow \textbf{55} & 74.\textbf{45} \longrightarrow 74.\textbf{5} \longrightarrow \textbf{75} \\
20.\textbf{2} \longrightarrow \textbf{20} & 42.\textbf{49} \longrightarrow 42.\textbf{5} \longrightarrow \textbf{43} \\
78.\textbf{1} \longrightarrow \textbf{78} & 36.\textbf{35} \longrightarrow 36.\textbf{4} \longrightarrow \textbf{36}
\end{array}
$$

When dividing, it is sometimes necessary to calculate as far as the **second** decimal fraction, as seen in some of the above examples, **when converting lb to kg.**

If there is any confusion concerning any of the conversions in this chapter, go back and review the calculations until they are well understood. Sometimes, it helps to read the information slowly and contemplate each point carefully. Also, sometimes the simplest math can be confusing: however, the purpose of this guide is to eliminate any confusion that may arise.

SUMMARY

When calculating drug dosages, there are only a **few** conversions that you as a paramedic or healthcare provider must be prepared to make in the field. As can be seen, it requires only **basic** math to do so. The most important concept to remember in the learning process is to **take your time and memorize each point before continuing on to the next.**

Review

Now that you feel comfortable with the conversion process, take your time and convert the following units of measure. Double check yourself to make sure you have placed the decimal point in its proper place.

UNIT 1: CONVERT THE FOLLOWING INTO MILLIGRAMS (mg)

1. .5 gm

2. .01 gm

3. 1.52 gm

4. .1 gm

5.   50 gm

6.   1 gm

7.   1.5 gm

8.   10 gm

9.   .001 gm

10. 2 gm

11. 25 gm

12. .25 gm

13. 2.5 gm

14. .025 gm

15. .0005 gm

16. .010 gm

17. .0010 gm

18. 1.25 gm

19. .00125 gm

20. 1.000 gm

21. 2.000 gm

22. .005 gm

23. .2 gm

24. .05 gm

25. 01.5 gm

UNIT 2: CONVERT THE FOLLOWING TO MICROGRAMS (µg)

1. .01 mg

2. .2 mg

3. 50.0 mg

4. 1.0 mg

5. 200 mg

6. 1.5 mg

7. 15 mg

8. .25 mg

9. .001 mg

10. 10 mg

11. 400 mg

12. .50 mg

13. .1 mg

14. 25 mg

15. .05 mg

16. 7.5 mg

17. 100 mg

18. .002 mg

19. .04 mg

20. 75 mg

21. 5 mg

22. 1 mg

23. .02 mg

24. 2.5 mg

25. 1.0 mg

UNIT 3: CONVERT THE FOLLOWING TO MILLILITERS (ml)

1. 1 L

2. .02 L

3. .25 L

4. .5 L

5. 2.5 L

6. .05 L

7. .001 L

8. 1.00 L

9. .75 L

10. .10 L

UNIT 4: CONVERT THE FOLLOWING TO CUBIC CENTIMETERS (cc's)

1. 500 ml

2. 1 ml

3. .5 ml

4. .25 ml

5. .1 ml

6. .04 ml

7. 2.5 ml

8. 1000 ml

9. 1.5 ml

10. 250 ml

UNIT 5: CONVERT THE FOLLOWING TO KILOGRAMS (kg)

1. 5 lb

2. 100 lb

3. 10 lb

4. 95 lb

5. 15 lb

6. 90 lb

7. 20 lb

8. 85 lb

9. 25 lb

10. 80 lb

11. 30 lb

12. 75 lb

13. 35 lb

Review

14. 70 lb

15. 40 lb

16. 65 lb

17. 45 lb

18. 60 lb

19. 50 lb

20. 55 lb

UNIT 6: CONVERT THE FOLLOWING TO KILOGRAMS (kg)

1. 110 lb

2. 300 lb

3. 120 lb

4. 290 lb

5. 130 lb

6. 280 lb

7.   140 lb

8.   270 lb

9.   150 lb

10.   260 lb

11.   160 lb

12.   250 lb

13.   170 lb

14.   240 lb

15.   180 lb

16.   230 lb

17.   190 lb

18.   **220 lb**

19.   200 lb

20.   210 lb

UNIT 7: CONVERT THE FOLLOWING TO KILOGRAMS (kg)

1. 88 lb

2. 142 lb

3. 9 lb

4. 285 lb

5. 6 lb

6. 278 lb

7. 68 lb

8. 243 lb

9. 128 lb

10. 183 lb

Answers

UNIT 1

1.   .5 gm ⟶ .5 0 0 = **500 mg**
                    1 2 3

2.   .01 gm ⟶ .0 1 0 = **10 mg**
                    1 2 3

3.   1.52 gm ⟶ 1.5 2 0 = **1520 mg**
                      1 2 3

4.   .1 gm ⟶ .1 0 0 = **100 mg**
                    1 2 3

5.   50 gm ⟶ 50.0 0 0 = **50,000 mg**
                      1 2 3

6.   1 gm ⟶ 1.0 0 0 = **1000 mg**
                    1 2 3

7.   1.5 gm ⟶ 1.5 0 0 = **1500 mg**
                      1 2 3

8.   10 gm ⟶ 10.0 0 0 = **10,000 mg**
                      1 2 3

9.   .001 gm ⟶ .0 0 1 = **1 mg**
                      1 2 3

10. 2 gm ⟶ 2.0̬0̬0̬ = **2000 mg**
     _{1 2 3}

11. 25 gm ⟶ 25.0̬0̬0̬ = **25,000 mg**
     _{1 2 3}

12. .25 gm ⟶ .2 5̬0̬ = **250 mg**
     _{1 2 3}

13. 2.5 gm ⟶ 2.5 0̬0̬ = **2500 mg**
     _{1 2 3}

14. .025 gm ⟶ .0 2̬ 5̬ = **25 mg**
     _{1 2 3}

15. .0005 gm ⟶ .0 0̬ 0̬ 5 = **.5 mg**
     _{1 2 3}

16. .010 gm ⟶ .0 1̬ 0̬ = **10 mg**
     _{1 2 3}

17. .0010 gm ⟶ .0 0̬ 1̬ 0 = **1.0 mg**
     _{1 2 3}

18. 1.25 gm ⟶ 1.2 5̬ 0̬ = **1250 mg**
     _{1 2 3}

19. .00125 gm ⟶ .0 0̬ 1̬ 2 5 = **1.25 mg**
     _{1 2 3}

20. 1.000 gm ⟶ 1.0̬0̬0̬ = **1000 mg**
     _{1 2 3}

21. 2.000 gm ⟶ 2.0̬0̬0̬ = **2000 mg**
     _{1 2 3}

22. .005 gm ⟶ .0 0̬ 5̬ = **5 mg**
     _{1 2 3}

23. .2 gm ⟶ .2̬0̬0̬ = **200 mg**
     _{1 2 3}

24. .05 gm ⟶ .0 5̬ 0̬ = **50 mg**
     _{1 2 3}

25. 01.5 gm ⟶ 01.5 0̬ 0̬ = **1500 mg**
     _{1 2 3}

UNIT 2

1. .01 mg ⟶ .0 1̬ 0̬ = **10 μg**
    _{1 2 3}

2. .2 mg ⟶ .2̬0̬0̬ = **200 μg**
    _{1 2 3}

3. 50.0 mg ⟶ 50.0̬0̬0̬ = **50,000 μg**
    _{1 2 3}

4. 1.0 mg ⟶ 1.0̬0̬0̬ = **1000 μg**
    _{1 2 3}

5. 200 mg $\longrightarrow$ 200.0 0 0 = **200,000 μg**

6. 1.5 mg $\longrightarrow$ 1.5 0 0 = **1500 μg**

7. 15 mg $\longrightarrow$ 15.0 0 0 = **15,000 μg**

8. .25 mg $\longrightarrow$ .2 5 0 = **250 μg**

9. .001 mg $\longrightarrow$ .0 0 1 = **1 μg**

10. 10 mg $\longrightarrow$ 10.0 0 0 = **10,000 μg**

11. 400 mg $\longrightarrow$ 400.0 0 0 = **400,000 μg**

12. .50 mg $\longrightarrow$ .5 0 0 = **500 μg**

13. .1 mg $\longrightarrow$ .1 0 0 = **100 μg**

14. 25 mg $\longrightarrow$ 25.0 0 0 = **25,000 μg**

15. .05 mg $\longrightarrow$ .0 5 0 = **50 μg**

16. 7.5 mg $\longrightarrow$ 7.5 0 0 = **7500 μg**

17. 100 mg $\longrightarrow$ 100.0 0 0 = **100,000 μg**

18. .002 mg $\longrightarrow$ .0 0 2 = **2 μg**

19. .04 mg $\longrightarrow$ .0 4 0 = **40 μg**

20. 75 mg $\longrightarrow$ 75.0 0 0 = **75,000 μg**

21. 5 mg $\longrightarrow$ 5.0 0 0 = **5000 μg**

22. 1 mg $\longrightarrow$ 1.0 0 0 = **1000 μg**

23. .02 mg $\longrightarrow$ .0 2 0 = **20 μg**

24. 2.5 mg $\longrightarrow$ 2.5 0 0 = **2500 μg**

25. **1.0 mg** $\longrightarrow$ 1.0 0 0 = **1000 μg**

Answers

UNIT 3

1. $1 \text{ L} \longrightarrow 1.\underset{1\ 2\ 3}{000} = $ **1000 ml**

2. $.02 \text{ L} \longrightarrow .\underset{1\ 2\ 3}{020} = $ **20 ml**

3. $.25 \text{ L} \longrightarrow .\underset{1\ 2\ 3}{250} = $ **250 ml**

4. **.5 L** $\longrightarrow .\underset{1\ 2\ 3}{500} = $ **500 ml**

5. $2.5 \text{ L} \longrightarrow 2.\underset{1\ 2\ 3}{500} = $ **2500 ml**

6. $.05 \text{ L} \longrightarrow .\underset{1\ 2\ 3}{050} = $ **50 ml**

7. $.001 \text{ L} \longrightarrow .\underset{1\ 2\ 3}{001} = $ **1 ml**

8. $1.00 \text{ L} \longrightarrow 1.\underset{1\ 2\ 3}{000} = $ **1000 ml**

9. $.75 \text{ L} \longrightarrow .\underset{1\ 2\ 3}{750} = $ **750 ml**

10. $.10 \text{ L} \longrightarrow .\underset{1\ 2\ 3}{100} = $ **100 ml**

UNIT 4

Recall that milliliters and cubic centimeters are interchangeable; therefore, no conversions are necessary.

1. 500 cc

2. 1 cc

3. .5 cc

4. .25 cc

5. .1 cc

6. .04 cc

7. 2.5 cc

8. 1000 cc

9. 1.5 cc

10. 250 cc

UNIT 5

1. 5 lb $\longrightarrow$ $2.2 \overline{)50}$ $2.2 \longrightarrow 2$

    Answer = 2 kg

2. 100 lb $\longrightarrow$ $2.2 \overline{)1000}$ $45.45 \longrightarrow 46$

    Answer = 46 kg

3. 10 lb $\longrightarrow$ $2.2 \overline{)100}$ $4.5 \longrightarrow 5$

    Answer = 5 kg

4. 95 lb $\longrightarrow$ $2.2 \overline{)950}$ $43.1 \longrightarrow 43$

    Answer = 43 kg

5. 15 lb $\longrightarrow$ $2.2 \overline{)150}$ $6.8 \longrightarrow 7$

    Answer = 7 kg

6. 90 lb $\longrightarrow$ $2.2 \overline{)900}$ $40.9 \longrightarrow 41$

    Answer = 41 kg

7. 20 lb $\longrightarrow$ $2.2 \overline{)200}$ 9.0

    Answer = 9 kg

8. 85 lb $\longrightarrow$ $2.2 \overline{)850}$ $38.6 \longrightarrow 39$

    Answer = 39 kg

9. 25 lb $\longrightarrow$ $2.2 \overline{)250}$ $11.3 \longrightarrow 11$

    Answer = 11 kg

10.   80 **lb** $\longrightarrow$ $2.2\overline{)800}$ $\dfrac{36.3}{}\longrightarrow 36$

Answer = 36 kg

11.   30 **lb** $\longrightarrow$ $2.2\overline{)300}$ $\dfrac{13.6}{}\longrightarrow 14$

Answer = 14 kg

12.   75 **lb** $\longrightarrow$ $2.2\overline{)750}$ $\dfrac{34.0}{}$

Answer = 34 kg

13.   35 **lb** $\longrightarrow$ $2.2\overline{)350}$ $\dfrac{15.9}{}\longrightarrow 16$

Answer = 16 kg

14.   70 **lb** $\longrightarrow$ $2.2\overline{)700}$ $\dfrac{31.8}{}\longrightarrow 32$

Answer = 32 kg

15.   40 **lb** $\longrightarrow$ $2.2\overline{)400}$ $\dfrac{18.1}{}\longrightarrow 18$

Answer = 18 kg

16.   65 **lb** $\longrightarrow$ $2.2\overline{)650}$ $\dfrac{29.5}{}\longrightarrow 30$

Answer = 30 kg

17.   45 **lb** $\longrightarrow$ $2.2\overline{)450}$ $\dfrac{20.45}{}\longrightarrow 21$

Answer = 21 kg

18.   60 **lb** $\longrightarrow$ $2.2\overline{)600}$ $\dfrac{27.2}{}\longrightarrow 27$

Answer = 27 kg

19.   50 **lb** $\longrightarrow$ $2.2\overline{)500}$ $\dfrac{22.7}{}\longrightarrow 23$

Answer = 23 kg

20.   55 **lb** $\longrightarrow$ $2.2\overline{)550}$ with quotient 25

Answer = 25 kg

UNIT 6

1.   110 **lb** $\longrightarrow$ $2.2\overline{)1100}$ with quotient 50

Answer = 50 kg

2.   300 **lb** $\longrightarrow$ $2.2\overline{)3000}$ with quotient 136.3 $\longrightarrow$ 136

Answer = 136 kg

3.   120 **lb** $\longrightarrow$ $2.2\overline{)1200}$ with quotient 54.5 $\longrightarrow$ 55

Answer = 55 kg

4.   290 **lb** $\longrightarrow$ $2.2\overline{)2900}$ with quotient 131.8 $\longrightarrow$ 132

Answer = 132 kg

5.   130 **lb** $\longrightarrow$ $2.2\overline{)1300}$ with quotient 59.0

Answer = 59 kg

6.   280 **lb** $\longrightarrow$ $2.2\overline{)2800}$ with quotient 127.2 $\longrightarrow$ 127

Answer = 127 kg

7.   140 **lb** $\longrightarrow$ $2.2\overline{)1400}$ with quotient 63.6 $\longrightarrow$ 64

Answer = 64 kg

8.   270 **lb** $\longrightarrow$ $2.2\overline{)2700}$ with quotient 122.7 $\longrightarrow$ 123

Answer = 123 kg

9.   150 **lb** $\longrightarrow$ $2.2\overline{)1500}$ with quotient 68.1 $\longrightarrow$ 68

Answer = 68 kg

10. $260 \text{ lb} \longrightarrow 2.2\overline{)2600} \quad \dfrac{118.1}{} \longrightarrow 118$

Answer = 118 kg

11. $160 \text{ lb} \longrightarrow 2.2\overline{)1600} \quad \dfrac{72.7}{} \longrightarrow 73$

Answer = 73 kg

12. $250 \text{ lb} \longrightarrow 2.2\overline{)2500} \quad \dfrac{113.6}{} \longrightarrow 114$

Answer = 114 kg

13. $170 \text{ lb} \longrightarrow 2.2\overline{)1700} \quad \dfrac{77.2}{} \longrightarrow 77$

Answer = 77 kg

14. $240 \text{ lb} \longrightarrow 2.2\overline{)2400} \quad \dfrac{109.0}{}$

Answer = 109 kg

15. $180 \text{ lb} \longrightarrow 2.2\overline{)1800} \quad \dfrac{81.8}{} \longrightarrow 82$

Answer = 82 kg

16. $230 \text{ lb} \longrightarrow 2.2\overline{)2300} \quad \dfrac{104.5}{} \longrightarrow 105$

Answer = 105 kg

17. $190 \text{ lb} \longrightarrow 2.2\overline{)1900} \quad \dfrac{86.3}{} \longrightarrow 86$

Answer = 86 kg

18. **220 lb** $\longrightarrow 2.2\overline{)2200} \quad \dfrac{100}{}$

Answer = 100 kg

19. $200 \text{ lb} \longrightarrow 2.2\overline{)2000} \quad \dfrac{90.9}{} \longrightarrow 91$

Answer = 91 kg

20.　210 **lb** $\longrightarrow$ $2.2\overline{\smash{)}2100}$ $\overset{95.45}{}\longrightarrow 96$

Answer = 96 kg

1.　88 **lb** $\longrightarrow$ $2.2\overline{\smash{)}880}$ $\overset{40}{}$

Answer = 40 kg

2.　142 **lb** $\longrightarrow$ $2.2\overline{\smash{)}1420}$ $\overset{64.5}{}\longrightarrow 65$

Answer = 65 kg

3.　9 **lb** $\longrightarrow$ $2.2\overline{\smash{)}90}$ $\overset{4.0}{}$

Answer = 4 kg

4.　285 **lb** $\longrightarrow$ $2.2\overline{\smash{)}2850}$ $\overset{129.5}{}\longrightarrow 130$

Answer = 130 kg

5.　6 **lb** $\longrightarrow$ $2.2\overline{\smash{)}60}$ $\overset{2.7}{}\longrightarrow 3$

Answer = 3 kg

6.　278 **lb** $\longrightarrow$ $2.2\overline{\smash{)}2780}$ $\overset{126.3}{}\longrightarrow 126$

Answer = 126 kg

7.　68 **lb** $\longrightarrow$ $2.2\overline{\smash{)}680}$ $\overset{30.9}{}\longrightarrow 31$

Answer = 31 kg

8.　243 **lb** $\longrightarrow$ $2.2\overline{\smash{)}2430}$ $\overset{110.45}{}\longrightarrow 111$

Answer = 111 kg

9.   128 **lb** $\longrightarrow$ $2.2\overline{\smash{)}1280}$ $58.1 \longrightarrow 58$

Answer = 58 kg

10.   183 **lb** $\longrightarrow$ $2.2\overline{\smash{)}1830}$ $83.1 \longrightarrow 83$

Answer = 83 kg

Chapter 1

Calculating the Desired Dose

IDENTIFYING THE DESIRED DOSE

Now that the method of conversions for the particular units of measure used in this guide have been established, the basic equation for calculating liquid drug administrations and dosages can be mastered. In this chapter, you will learn to **identify** the desired dose, part of the first step of this four-step formula.

STEP 1

Establish the desired dose (DD). **DD is defined as the amount of a particular drug to be administered.** When an order has been given either verbally, by protocol, or other means, you must **first** be able to **identify** the desired dose and separate it from the other information given. At times it becomes necessary to calculate the desired dose, as explained further in this chapter.

NOTE: A slash (/) is the symbol for the word **per** as illustrated below. See examples:

2 mg/min	Reads:	2 milligrams **per** minute
5 µg/kg/min	Reads:	5 micrograms **per** kilogram per minute
5 mg/2 cc	Reads:	5 milligrams **per** 2 cubic centimeters
1 mg/10 cc	Reads:	1 milligram **per** 10 cubic centimeters

The desired dose is simply the **amount** or **quantity** of the physician's order. Sometimes the amount involves a time factor; however, more commonly it is just the quantity as a single dose. See examples:

An ED physician orders **.3 mg** of epinephrine 1:1000 to be given sq. On hand is an ampule containing 1 mg in 1 cc. What is the desired dose **(DD)**?

STEP 1   DD = .3 mg

According to protocol, you must administer **2 mg** of Narcan IV. On hand is a vial containing 2 mg in 2 cc. What is the desired dose **(DD)**?

STEP 1   DD = 2 mg

While en route to the hospital with a cardiac patient, the physician orders you to start a Lidocaine drip to be run at **2 mg/min.** On hand is a vial containing 1 gm of Lidocaine, a 250 cc bag of normal saline, and a minidrip administration set. What is the desired dose **(DD)**?

STEP 1   DD = 2 mg/min

Note the time factor in the physician's order of 2 mg **per min**.

CALCULATING THE DESIRED DOSE

Sometimes, in reference to the desired dose, it becomes necessary not only to **identify** the desired dose but also to **calculate** it, as can be seen in the following examples:

You have been ordered to initiate a dopamine **drip** to be run at **5 μg/kg/min.** The patient weighs **175** pounds. On hand are two ampules containing 200 mg of dopamine in each, a 500 cc bag of normal saline, and a minidrip administration set. What is the desired dose **(DD)**?

Remember, in this particular question, the order is 5 μg/**kg**/min. Take note that the order of 5 μg is **per** kg. The patient's weight is **175** pounds. The pounds must **first** be converted into **kg, then** the **5 μg** must be **multiplied** by the total number of **kg** to obtain the desired dose. See example:

$$\text{First: } 2.2 \overline{)1750} \quad \frac{79.5 \longrightarrow 80 \text{ kg}}{} \qquad \textbf{Then: } 80 \times 5 \text{ μg} = 400 \text{ μg}$$

DD = 400 μg/min

Recall that when calculating **kg**, if the answer includes a decimal fraction, it is acceptable to **round off** to the nearest **whole number** (Refer to the introduction on converting lb to kg). Multiplying the kg times the desired dosage which is per kg will result in the elimination of the word kg from the desired dose, leaving only 400 **μg/min** as the desired dose. After this step in the formula, the patient's weight is then **no** longer necessary in the calculation process.

You have been ordered to give **2 μg/kg/min** of dopamine via **drip.** The patient's weight is estimated at **220** pounds. On hand is a 10 cc vial containing 400 mg of dopamine, a 250 cc bag of normal saline, and a minidrip administration set. What is the desired dose **(DD)**?

$$\text{First: } 2.2\overline{)2200} \quad \begin{array}{c} 100 \textbf{ kg} \end{array} \qquad \textbf{Then: } 100 \times 2 \text{ μg} = 200 \text{ μg}$$

$$\textbf{DD} = \textbf{200 μg/min}$$

All too often, class, state, and national exams tend to provide you with more information than you actually need. For example:

You have been ordered to initiate a drip to be run at 10 μg/min **with a patient weight of 150 pounds.** On hand is a prefilled syringe containing 1 mg, a 250 cc bag of solution, and a minidrip administration set. What is the desired dose **(DD)**?

$$\textbf{DD} = \textbf{10 μg/min}$$

As you can see, you have been ordered to give 10 μg**/min.** Per **kg** is **not** even mentioned in the order. Therefore, the patient's weight is **irrelevant** in this particular problem. So when you run across this particular circumstance, you will know that they are merely trying to *throw you off* by providing you with the patient's weight.

Selecting and then calculating the desired dose can be simple. At this point, if there is any confusion whatsoever, go back and review the chapter. It is very important that you **clearly** understand each step before continuing on to the next.

SUMMARY

As a paramedic or healthcare provider, you must be able to recognize the desired dose. Sometimes it may become necessary to calculate the patient's weight in order to administer proper dosages. As you have learned, **only basic math skills are required for this simple step.** Thus, the first step of the easy 4-step formula is:

STEP 1   DD

Review

Below are some practice questions that should assist you in mastering the first step of this formula. You should now be able to identify not only the desired dose but also be able to calculate it when necessary. Keep in mind that sometimes there may be additional information provided that may not necessarily be needed in order to calculate **Step 1** of this formula.

1. You have been ordered by the physician to administer 75 mg of Lidocaine IV. On hand, you have a prefilled syringe containing 100 mg in 5 cc. What is the desired dose?

2. You are ordered to give 1 mEq/**kg** of sodium bicarbonate (Na HCO$_3$) via IO route. The patient is a 6-month-old weighing 15 pounds. What is the desired dose?

3. You are ordered to give 3 μg/**kg/min** of dopamine by IV **drip.** The patient weighs 185 pounds. On hand, you have two vials of Dopamine containing 200 mg/5 cc each, a 250 cc bag of normal saline, and a minidrip administration set. What is the desired dose?

4. On scene, you have a patient requiring, according to protocol, 2.5 mg of Valium IV. You estimate the patient's weight at 200 pounds. On hand, you have a prefilled syringe containing 10 mg/5 cc. What is the desired dose?

5. You have a patient in cardiac arrest showing V-fib on the monitor. The ED physician has ordered the administration of 300 mg of amiodarone (Cordarone) IV. Your patient weighs 190 pounds. What is the desired dose?

6. You have been ordered to administer 1 mg/**kg** of Lidocaine IV to a 6-year-old child. The parent states that her child weighs 46 pounds. What is the desired dose?

7. For the preceeding 6-year-old patient, the physician has requested that you follow up with a Lidocaine **drip** to be run at 20 μg/**kg/min.** Keep in mind that your patient's weight is 46 pounds. What is the desired dose?

8. While assisting the ED staff, the physician has ordered you to administer .02 mg/**kg** of atropine IV to an 18-month-old male weighing 24 pounds. What is the desired dose?

9. According to protocol, you must immediately administer 6 mg of adenosine rapid IV push to your patient weighing 150 pounds. What is the desired dose?

10. While en route to the hospital with your 3-year-old patient, medical control has ordered you to administer .01 mg/**kg** of epinephrine 1:10,000 IV. The patient's weight is 34 pounds. What is the desired dose?

Answers

1. STEP 1   **DD = 75 mg**

2. STEP 1   DD = 1 mEq/kg $\longrightarrow$ $2.2\overline{)150}$ $\begin{array}{c}6.8\end{array}$ $\longrightarrow$ **7 kg**

   $\longrightarrow$ 7 × 1 mEq = 7 mEq

   DD = 7 mEq

3. STEP 1   DD = 3 μg/kg/min $\longrightarrow$ $2.2\overline{)1850}$ $\begin{array}{c}84\ \textbf{kg}\end{array}$

   $\longrightarrow$ 84 × 3 μg = 252 μg

   DD = 252 μg/min

4. STEP 1   **DD = 2.5 mg**

5. STEP 1   **DD = 300 mg**

   Recall the ED physician did not order the Cordarone per kg. Therefore, the patient's weight is not relevant in this question.

6. STEP 1   DD = 1 mg/kg   ⟶ $2.2\overline{)460}$ $\dfrac{20.9}{}$ ⟶ 21 **kg**

                 ⟶ 21 × 1 mg = 21 mg

            DD = 21 mg

7. STEP 1   DD = 20 μg/kg/min   ⟶ $2.2\overline{)460}$ $\dfrac{20.9}{}$ ⟶ 21 **kg**

                 ⟶ 21 × 20 μg = 420 μg

            DD = 420 μg/min

8. STEP 1   DD = .02 mg/kg   ⟶ $2.2\overline{)240}$ $\dfrac{10.9}{}$ ⟶ 11 **kg**

                 ⟶ 11 × .02 mg = .22 mg

            DD = .22 mg

9. STEP 1   **DD = 6 mg**

10. STEP 1   DD = .01 mg/kg   ⟶ $2.2\overline{)340}$ $\dfrac{15.45}{}$ ⟶ 16 **kg**

                 ⟶ 16 × .01 mg = .16 mg

            DD = .16 mg

Chapter 2

Calculating the Concentration

LEARNING THE FORMULA

Now that you have mastered the ability to identify the desired dose and to perform the necessary calculations involved, the formula for **calculating the concentration** of drugs supplied in vials, ampules, prefilled syringes, and premixed bags can be established.

STEP 2

> Calculate the concentration (C) of the drug being administered. The concentration is the **total** weight of the drug (normally gm, mg, μg, and units) mixed in the total amount of **cc's** (ml).

When performing this step, always remember that the concentration is calculated by placing weight **over** cc's **(mg/cc).** When setting up the formula, always make sure that it is weight/cc. Many times people tend to get this reversed by placing the cc's over the weight, thus getting an incorrect answer along with extreme confusion during the calculation process.

The easiest way to remember this is to imagine a diver (weight) jumping into the water (cc's). Thus, the diver (weight) is on the top and the water (cc's) is on the bottom. The concentration is normally found located on the label of each container, whether it be an ampule, vial, prefilled syringe, or a premixed bag. In most cases, the **concentration** is expressed as **mg/cc** or mg/ml. Sometimes, in multidose containers, the concentration is not broken down into how many mg's there are **per** cc. See examples:

| 1 mg**/10** cc | 2 mg**/2** cc | 50 mg**/2** cc | 200 mg**/250** cc | 1 gm**/250** cc |

Throughout this guide, the **concentration** will be expressed as **mg/cc** or mg/ml. Keep a mental note that cc's and ml's are interchangeable. When another weight or measurement other than mg is indicated, such as gm or μg, simply substitute that measurement.

It becomes necessary to divide the **total** number of **mg's** by the **total** number of **cc's** in order to obtain how many mg's there are per **each** cc. See example:

$$2 \textbf{ mg/2 cc} \quad \text{or} \quad 2\overline{)2}^{\,1} = 1 \text{ mg/\textbf{cc}}$$

When calculating the concentration, keep in mind that you are **only** dividing the numbers, **not** the measurements. The **mg's** will remain on the **top** and the **cc's** will remain on the **bottom.** See example:

$$2 \textbf{ mg/2 cc} = 1 \textbf{ mg/cc}$$

Only the numbers change due to the division process. According to basic algebra, note that in the above example, after breaking the concentration down to 1 mg per **cc,** the number 1 is not written down preceding the cc. Thus, it is taken that this is an invisible number 1. See example:

$$1 \text{ mg/}\textbf{(1)} \text{ cc} = 1 \text{ mg/cc}$$

The example of 200 mg/250 cc, which was shown earlier in this unit, can be rewritten to be **250 $\overline{)}$200.** The divisor is **250,** and the dividend is **200.** By dividing the 200 by 250, the answer will acquire a decimal fraction because the divisor of 250 is larger than the dividend of 200. During this division process, it becomes necessary to **add** a zero to that dividend. See example:

$$250\overline{)200.0}^{\,.}$$

Before adding a zero to the dividend to complete the division process, be sure to place the decimal at the **end** of the **whole number** and in the **answer space,** as shown in the above example.

Note what occurred with the decimal point in the previous example. The decimal does **not** move since the divisor of 250 did not contain a decimal fraction, so the decimal will remain in the same location in the answer as it is in the dividend. Whenever the denominator **(bottom number)** is larger than the numerator (top number), as it is in 200 mg/**250** cc, it is automatically taken that the answer will be a decimal fraction. See example:

$$200\ \text{mg}/\mathbf{250}\ \text{cc} \qquad \text{or} \qquad 250\overline{)200.0}^{\,.8}$$

Prior to dividing, realize that the answer will be a decimal fraction. You can then calculate your answer, and if it is not a decimal fraction, you will know the equation has been set up incorrectly (note the above example). Using the answer of **.8** in the above example, it sometimes becomes necessary to convert the **.8** mg to μg's. If your desired dose is in another measurement, as seen in the desired dose of 5 **μg**/min, you must then convert the mg to μg, by moving the decimal three places to the right (as noted in the introduction on converting mg to μg). See example:

$$.8\underset{1\ 2\ 3}{0\,0} = 800\ \mathbf{\mu g}/\text{cc}$$

Sometimes it is necessary to convert mg to μg **before** calculating the concentration. For example, when calculating the concentration for a drip, the drug comes supplied in a prefilled syringe containing 1 mg. You mix that into a bag of 250 cc. To avoid working with decimals at this point with this particular drip, it is much easier to convert the 1 **mg** to **1000** μg and then calculate your concentration. See example:

$$1\ \mathbf{mg}/250\ \text{cc} \longrightarrow 1\underset{1\ 2\ 3}{0\,0\,0}\ \mathbf{\mu g}/250\ \text{cc} = 4\ \mu g/\text{cc}$$

Instead of:

$$1\ \text{mg}/250\ \text{cc} \longrightarrow .0\underset{1\ 2\ 3}{0\,4} = 4\ \mu g/\text{cc}$$

Remember, whatever **measurement** is used in the desired dose, it must be **reflected** in the end result of the calculated concentration. See examples:

You have been ordered to give 25 **mg** of a particular drug that is supplied in 50 mg/5 cc. What is the concentration (**C**)?

STEP 1   DD = 25 **mg**

STEP 2   C = 50 mg/5 cc   or $5\overline{)50}^{\,10} = 10\ \mathbf{mg}/\text{cc}$

You have been ordered to start a drip to be run at 10 **μg**/min. On hand you have 1 **mg** of a given drug and a 250 cc bag of solution. What is the concentration (**C**)?

Note: In this problem, you must convert the one **mg** to **μg's** since the desired dose is in **μg's.**

STEP 1   DD = 10 **μg**/min

STEP 2   C = 1 **mg**/250 cc ⟶ $\dfrac{1000 \text{ μg}}{250 \text{ cc}}$ = 4 **μg**/cc

---

You have received an order for 20 mg of Lasix IV. On hand is a vial with 4 cc containing 40 mg. What is the concentration (**C**)?

Note: When calculating the concentration, always place **mg's** over **cc's.**

STEP 1   DD = 20 **mg**

STEP 2   C = 40 **mg**/4 **cc**   or $4\overline{)40}$ $\overset{10}{}$ = 10 **mg**/cc

---

You have been ordered to give .3 mg of epinephrine IV. The drug comes supplied in an ampule with 1 cc containing 1 mg. What is the concentration (**C**)?

STEP 1   DD = .3 mg
STEP 2   **C = 1 mg/cc**

Note: In the above problem, the concentration is already given in its most condensed form. Therefore, there was no calculating to be done; only identifying the concentration was necessary.

When calculating the concentration of a bag with drug additives to be used for an **IV drip** administration, the volume (or amount of cc's) in the ampule, vial, or prefilled syringe is **not** to be used in the calculation of this step. **Again,** this rule only applies to IV drips. However, the cc's in the container into which the drug is being mixed (usually a bag or a bottle) is the amount that you use for calculating the concentration. In reference to calculating drips on exams, the amount of cc's in an ampule, vial, or prefilled syringe is normally not given, only the amounts of cc's in the bag, such as 50 cc, 100 cc, 250 cc, 500 cc, or 1000 cc. See example:

You have been ordered to start a dopamine drip to be run at 4 μg/kg/min. On hand is a vial containing 200 mg, a **250 cc bag** of normal saline, and a minidrip tubing. Your patient's weight is 150 pounds. What is the concentration (**C**)?

STEP 1   DD = 4 **μg**/kg/min ⟶ $2.2\overline{)1500}$ $\overset{68 \text{ kg}}{}$

⟶ 68 × 4 **μg** = 272 **μg**
DD = 272 **μg**/min

STEP 2   C = $\dfrac{200 \text{ mg}}{250 \text{ cc}}$ = .8 mg/cc ⟶ .800 = **800 μg/cc**

Again, when dealing with a drip problem, normally the only cc's to be used in the calculation are those in the bag.

SUMMARY

Up to this point, you have learned to **identify** the desired dose, how to calculate the desired dose, and how to calculate the concentration. Thus, the first two steps of this easy four-step formula are:

STEP 1   **DD**

STEP 2   **C** (always weight/cc)
                    e.g.—**mg/cc**

Review

Provided below are some practice questions to apply what has been learned in Chapter 1, on calculating the desired dose, and in this chapter, on calculating the concentration. Some of the answers may appear obvious to you, but it is necessary that you calculate each step.

1. The doctor has ordered you to give **20 mg** of **Lasix IV.** On hand you have a vial containing **40 mg** in **4 cc.**
   a. What is the DD?   **b.** What is the C?

2. You have been ordered to give **8 mg** of **Decadron** IV. On hand is a vial containing **20 mg** in **5 cc.**
   a. What is the DD?　　　　　　　　**b.** What is the C?

3. You have been ordered to give **2.5 mg** of **Valium** IV. On hand is a pre-filled syringe containing **10 mg** in **2 cc.**
   a. What is the DD?　　　　　　　　**b.** What is the C?

4. While on scene, you are unable to establish an IV access on your 6-year-old patient. The **blood glucose** level is **30.** Your patient weighs about **45** pounds. Per protocol, you must administer **.025 mg/kg** of **Glucagon** IM. On hand is a vial containing **1 mg** of **Glucagon** in powder form and another vial containing **1 cc** of bacteriostatic water to be used for the dilution of the **Glucagon.**
   a. What is the DD?　　　　　　　　**b.** What is the C?

5. You have been ordered to initiate a **dopamine drip.** Your order is to give **5 μg/kg/min.** Your patient's weight is **200** pounds. On hand are two ampules containing **200 mg** in **each,** a **250 cc** bag of normal saline, and a **60 gtt** administration set.

    Note: On hand are two ampules. Be sure to use the total amount of drug supplied in the problem.
    a. What is the DD?   b. What is the C?

6. The physician has ordered you to administer **.5 mg** of **Stadol** IV. The drug comes supplied in a **2 cc** vial containing **2 mg.**
    a. What is the DD?   b. What is the C?

7. The ED physician has ordered you to start an IV **drip** to be run at **10 μg/min.** On hand is a prefilled syringe containing **1 mg** in 5 cc, a **250 cc** bag of solution, and a minidrip set. The doctor has informed you that your patient only weighs 150 pounds.
    a. What is the DD?   b. What is the C?

8. You have been ordered to give **25 mg** of **diphenhydramine** IM. On hand is a prefilled tubex containing **50 mg** in **1 cc.**
   a. What is the DD?   **b.** What is the C?

9. The on-call physician orders **.5 mg** of **epinephrine 1:10,000** solution to be given IVP. On hand, you have a prefilled syringe containing **1 mg** in **10 cc.**
   a. What is the DD?   **b.** What is the C?

10. According to protocol, you must administer **.4 mg** of **naloxone** IV. On hand is an ampule with **2 cc** containing **2 mg.**
    a. What is the DD?   **b.** What is the C?

Answer

1. **a.** STEP 1   DD = **20 mg**

   b. STEP 2   C = 40 mg/4 cc   or $4\overline{)40}$ $\dfrac{10}{} =$ **10 mg/cc**

2. **a.** STEP 1   DD = **8 mg**

   b. STEP 2   C = 20 mg/5 cc   or $5\overline{)20}$ $\dfrac{4}{} =$ **4 mg/cc**

3. **a.** STEP 1   DD = **2.5 mg**

   b. STEP 2   C = 10 mg/2 cc   or $2\overline{)10}$ $\dfrac{5}{} =$ **5 mg/cc**

4. **a.** STEP 1   DD = .025 mg/kg ⟶ $2.2\overline{)450}$ $\dfrac{20.45}{} \longrightarrow$ **21 kg**

                               ⟶ 21 × .025 mg = .525

                               ⟶ .5 mg

                     DD = **.5 mg**

   Since the patient's weight is **estimated** at 45 pounds, the actual answer of **.525** can safely be rounded down to **.5 mg**.

b. STEP 2   C = **1 mg/1 cc**

After drawing the 1 cc from the vial and mixing it into the 1 mg vial of powder, the two mixed together already contain the most condensed concentration of **1 mg per cc.** Therefore, no calculation is necessary for this step.

5.   **a.** STEP 1 $DD = 5\ \mu g/kg/min \longrightarrow 2.2\overline{)2000}$ $\dfrac{90.9 \longrightarrow 91\ \textbf{kg}}{}$

$$\longrightarrow 91 \times 5\ \mu g = 455\ \mu g$$

$$DD = \textbf{455}\ \boldsymbol{\mu} \textbf{g/min}$$

b. STEP 2 $C = 400\ mg/250\ cc$ or $250\overline{)400.0}$ $\dfrac{1.6 = 1.6\ mg/cc}{}$

$$\longrightarrow 1.6\ mg \longrightarrow 1\,6\,0\,0.\mu g = \textbf{1600}\ \boldsymbol{\mu}\textbf{g/cc}$$

6.   **a.** STEP 1 $DD = \textbf{.5 mg}$

b. STEP 2 $C = \textbf{2 mg/2 cc}$ or $2\overline{)2}$ $\dfrac{1 = \textbf{1 mg/cc}}{}$

7.   **a.** STEP 1 $DD = \textbf{10}\ \boldsymbol{\mu}\textbf{g/min}$

b. STEP 2 $C = 1\ mg/250\ cc \longrightarrow 1\,0\,0\,0\ \mu g/250\ cc$ or $250\overline{)1000}$ $\dfrac{4}{}$

$$\textbf{Answer} = \textbf{4}\ \boldsymbol{\mu}\textbf{g/cc}$$

8.   **a.** STEP 1 $DD = \textbf{25 mg}$

b. STEP 2 $C = \textbf{50 mg/cc}$

9.   **a.** STEP 1 $DD = \textbf{.5 mg}$

b. STEP 2 $C = 1\ mg/10\ cc$ or $10\overline{)1.0}$ $\dfrac{.1 = \textbf{.1 mg/cc}}{}$

10.   **a.** STEP 1 $DD = \textbf{.4 mg}$

b. STEP 2 $C = 2\ mg/2\ cc$ or $2\overline{)2}$ $\dfrac{1 = \textbf{1 mg/cc}}{}$

Chapter 3

Calculating the cc's

LEARNING THE FORMULA

Now that the first two steps of this formula have been learned—identifying and calculating the desired dose, and calculating the concentration—we can proceed to the third step.

STEP 3

Calculate the amount of cc's to be delivered. There are two purposes for this particular calculation: (1) when giving a drug through **SQ, IM, IV, ET,** or **IO** it is necessary to calculate the amount of cc's to be drawn from a particular container (ampule or vial) or to be pushed through a prefilled syringe so that the desired dose can be delivered, or (2) to calculate the amount of cc's needed to figure gtts/min, which is required in step 4, on calculating drip rates. For whichever reason cc's are being calculated, the formula is:

$$\frac{DD}{C}$$

If the route of administration is SQ, IM, ET, IO push, or IVP, only the first three steps of this formula, (1) DD, (2) C, and (3) DD/C, need to be calculated, eliminating step 4, which is defined in chapter 4. The reason for eliminating step 4 when the route of administration is SQ, IM, ET, IO push, or IVP is that ultimately you need to calculate only the number of cc's to draw from a given container, not the drops per minute, as required for a drip administration. If a prefilled syringe is being used, it is necessary to calculate only the number of cc's to push from the syringe.

This step can be very simple because all it involves is dividing the desired dose by the concentration. See example:

$$C \overline{)DD} \qquad \text{or} \qquad \frac{DD}{C}$$

When dealing with this step, many times there are several **zeros** in these numbers. See example:

$$\frac{DD}{C} = \frac{500 \text{ mg}}{50 \text{ mg/cc}}$$

To simplify the division process in the above example, some zeros can be **canceled out.** When canceling zeros, the **same** number of zeros must be canceled in both the numerator (top number) **and** denominator (bottom number). See example:

$$\frac{DD}{C} = \frac{50\cancel{0} \text{ mg}}{5\cancel{0} \text{ mg/cc}} = \frac{50 \text{ mg}}{5 \text{ mg/cc}}$$

In the above example, **one** zero was able to be canceled in both the numerator of **500** and the denominator of **50.** Another example of canceling out zeros follows:

$$\frac{DD}{C} = \frac{50\cancel{00} \text{ mg}}{5\cancel{00} \text{ mg/cc}} = \frac{50 \text{ mg}}{5 \text{ mg/cc}}$$

In this last example, **two** zeros were able to be canceled in both the numerator and the denominator.

Because zeros can be canceled out, **measurements** also can be canceled. See example:

$$\frac{DD}{C} = \frac{50 \cancel{mg}}{5 \cancel{mg}/cc} = 10 \text{ cc}$$

After canceling the mg's, the **only** measurement left is **cc.** So the answer will be in cc's, as noted in the previous example.

Following are a few examples on the calculations involved in step 3.

You have been ordered to give **2.5 mg** of **valium.** On hand is a vial with **2 cc** containing **10 mg**. How many **cc's** would you draw?

STEP 1   DD = **2.5 mg**

STEP 2 $C = \dfrac{10 \text{ mg}}{2 \text{ cc}} = $ **5 mg/cc**

STEP 3 $\dfrac{\textbf{DD}}{\textbf{C}} = \dfrac{2.5 \text{ mg}}{5 \text{ mg/cc}}$ or $5\overline{)2.5}^{\,.5} = $ **.5 cc**

Explanation: **First** you identified the desired dose, which was **2.5** mg. **Then,** in step 2, you calculated the concentration by dividing 10 mg by 2 cc (remember, mg over cc **[mg/cc]** when calculating the concentration), leaving **5 mg/cc.** Then, in step **3,** the desired dose of 2.5 mg was divided by the concentration of 5 mg/cc. So 2.5 mg divided by 5 mg/cc equals **.5 cc** (remember that the mg's canceled), leaving **cc** as the only measurement.

You have been ordered to give **1 mg/kg** of **Lidocaine** IV. Your patient weighs **150** pounds. The prefilled syringe contains **100 mg** in **5 cc.** How many **cc's** will you push?

STEP 1   DD = 1 mg/kg $2.2\overline{)1500}^{\,68 \textbf{ kg}}$ 68 × 1 mg = 68 mg

DD = **68 mg**

STEP 2 $C = \dfrac{100 \text{ mg}}{5 \text{ cc}} = $ **20 mg/cc**

STEP 3 $\dfrac{\textbf{DD}}{\textbf{C}} = \dfrac{68 \text{ mg}}{20 \text{ mg/cc}} = $ **3.4 cc**

Explanation: In the previous example, the desired dose was ordered **per** kg. So, **first** the pounds were **converted** to kg (by dividing the 150 pounds by **2.2**), leaving an answer of **68 kg.** You then **multiplied** the total number of **kg,** which was 68, by the **desired dose** per kg, which was 1 mg **per** kg, leaving a desired dose of **68 mg.** In step **2,** you calculated the **concentration** by dividing the number of mg's by the number of cc's of the on-hand drug, which was supplied in a prefilled syringe. In step **3,** you divided the **desired dose** by the **concentration.** The mg's canceled out, leaving you with **3.4 cc** to push from the prefilled syringe.

The physician has ordered **20 mg** of **Lasix** IV. On hand is a vial with **4 cc** containing **40 mg.** How many **cc's** will you give?

STEP 1   DD = **20 mg**

STEP 2 $C = \dfrac{40 \text{ mg}}{4 \text{ cc}} = $ **10 mg/cc**

STEP 3 $\dfrac{\textbf{DD}}{\textbf{C}} = \dfrac{20 \text{ mg}}{10 \text{ mg/cc}} = $ **2 cc**

Explanation: **First** you identified the desired dose of 20 mg. In step **2,** you took your on-hand medication supplied in the vial and divided the **mg's** by the **cc's.** In step **3,** you divided the **desired dose** by the **concentration.** The mg's **canceled,** leaving an answer of **2 cc.** This amount would then be drawn from the vial and administered to your patient.

THE TIME FACTOR

Note that when a **drip** has been indicated for a particular drug administration, the desired dose will be ordered over a certain **time** frame, normally per minute. See examples:

$$2 \text{ mg/\textbf{min}} \qquad \text{or} \qquad 10 \text{ μg/kg/\textbf{min}}$$

You should **never** leave out any part of the problem to "cut corners" when calculating on paper. Consistently **label** each number or figure accordingly. See examples:

$$\frac{\textbf{DD}}{\textbf{C}} = \frac{20 \text{ mg}}{10 \text{ mg/cc}}$$

$$\frac{\textbf{DD}}{\textbf{C}} = \frac{2 \text{ mg/min}}{4 \text{ mg/cc}}$$

$$\textbf{DD} = 2 \text{ mg/min}$$
$$\textbf{DD} = 10 \text{ μg/kg/min}$$

$$\textbf{C} = 4 \text{ mg/cc}$$
$$\textbf{C} = 800 \text{ μg/cc}$$

Never leave out any measurements or time factors. Failure to include any identifying factors, such as DD =, C =, DD/C =, mg's, cc's, or minutes, will only confuse and complicate the calculation learning process.

Concerning **step 3** of this formula on calculating cc's, if a **time factor** has been given in the desired dose, be sure to always include it throughout each step, especially this one. But don't let the time factor confuse you, because it has absolutely nothing to do with the calculation of this step. However, it has everything to do with **step 4.** This is why it is so important not to leave this **factor** out at any time throughout your calculations.

Again, be sure to place it **(min)** properly in the equation, but disregard it when figuring your math through step 3. See example:

$$
\begin{array}{ll}
\text{STEP 1} & \text{DD} = 2 \text{ mg/\textbf{min}} \\
\text{STEP 2} & \text{C} = 4 \text{ mg/cc} \\
\text{STEP 3} & \dfrac{\text{DD}}{\text{C}} = \dfrac{2 \text{ mg/\textbf{min}}}{4 \text{ mg/cc}} = .5 \text{ cc/\textbf{min}}
\end{array}
$$

In reference to the preceding example, **cc's** is the only measurement left after canceling the **mg's.** The time factor **always** goes on the **bottom** of any **answer** throughout any equation. See example:

$$\frac{\text{DD}}{\text{C}} = \frac{(\text{Top}) \, 2 \text{ mg/\textbf{min}} \, (\textbf{bottom})}{4 \text{ mg/cc}} = (\text{Top}) \, .5 \text{ cc/\textbf{min}} \, (\textbf{bottom})$$

Since the **minute** is part of the desired dose, it must **remain** with the desired dose, as noted in 2 mg/min, until you have calculated the answer in step **3** of the formula. The time factor then **moves** to the bottom in the **answer** in step **3**, as shown previously in **.5 cc/min.**

When calculating **cc's** to further be used in the calculation of step 4, your answer will usually involve **decimal fractions,** especially in drips such as Dopamine. When this is the case, it is necessary that you divide only to the nearest 1000th, which is the **third** decimal fraction (**.222**). Rounding off to the nearest whole number is not suggested at this point when working with drip calculations. See examples:

$$\frac{DD}{C} = \frac{150 \text{ μg/min}}{800 \text{ μg/cc}} = .187 \text{ cc/min} \qquad \frac{DD}{C} = \frac{340 \text{ μg/min}}{1600 \text{ μg/cc}} = .212 \text{ cc/min}$$

SUMMARY

Just as you have learned, the third step of this process consists simply of dividing the desired dose **by** the concentration. Always remember to **label** figures and equations and don't **"cut corners."** This will only confuse you. So far, three of the four steps consists of:

STEP 1   **DD**

STEP 2   **C** (always weight/cc)

             e.g.—**mg/cc**

STEP 3 $\dfrac{DD}{C}$

Review

Following are a few practice questions pertaining to step 3. Simply complete the first three steps of the formula that you have learned so far. Remember, some of the answers may seem obvious to you, but it would be very much to your advantage to work out each and every step.

1. An order has been given for a particular **drip** delivering **10 μg/min.** On hand is **1 mg,** a **250 cc** bag of fluid, and a minidrip administration set. How many **cc's** per minute must be delivered to give the DD?

2. You have been ordered to give **8 mg** of **Decadron** IV. On hand, you have a **5 cc** vial containing **20 mg.** How many **cc's** must you draw to give your DD?

3. A physician has given you an order for a **Lidocaine drip** to be run at **2 mg/min.** On hand are **two grams** of **Lidocaine,** a **500 cc** bag of normal saline, and a minidrip administration set. How many **cc's** per **minute** must be delivered to give the DD?

4. The doctor has ordered you to give **25 mg** of **diphenhydramine** IV. On hand is a **2 cc** vial containing **50 mg.** How many **cc's** must you draw to give the DD?

5. You are at the residence of a patient who requires a **dopamine drip.** Your protocol states to give **2 μg/kg/min.** Your patient weighs **220** pounds. On hand is **400 mg** of **dopamine,** a **500 cc** bag of normal saline, and a minidrip administration set. How many **cc's** per **minute** must be delivered in order to give the DD?

6. You are on scene with a 1-year-old male requiring **1 mg/kg** of **Lidocaine** IV. The mother advises you that her son weighs **22** pounds. Your Lidocaine comes supplied in a prefilled syringe containing **100 mg** in **5 ml.** How many **ml's** would you administer?

7. You have been ordered to give **12 mg** of **Decadron** IV. On hand is a vial containing **20 mg** in **5 cc.** How many **cc's** would you give?

8. You are en route to the hospital and your patient requires **6 mg** of **adenosine** rapid IVP. On hand is a **2 cc** vial containing **6 mg.** How many **cc's** would you draw?

9. A **dopamine drip** has been ordered to be run at **8 μg/kg/min.** On hand is a vial containing **400 mg,** a **250 cc** bag of normal saline, and a minidrip. If your patient's weight is **145** pounds, how many **cc's** per **minute** would you deliver?

10. A **Lidocaine drip** has been ordered to be run at **3 mg/min.** On hand you have a vial containing **1 gm,** a **250 cc** bag of normal saline, and a minidrip. If your patient weighs **220** pounds, how many **cc's** per **minute** do you need to give?

Answers

1. STEP 1   DD = **10 μg/min**

   STEP 2   C = 1 mg/250 cc $\longrightarrow$ 1 $\underset{1\ 2\ 3}{000}$ μg/250 cc = **4 μg/cc**

   STEP 3 $\dfrac{DD}{C} = \dfrac{10\ \cancel{μg}/min}{4\ \cancel{μg}/cc}$ = **2.5 cc/min**

2. STEP 1   DD = **8 mg**

   STEP 2   C = 20 mg/5 cc = **4 mg/cc**

   STEP 3 $\dfrac{DD}{C} = \dfrac{8\ \cancel{mg}}{4\ \cancel{mg}/cc}$ = **2 cc**

3. STEP 1   DD = **2 mg/min**

   STEP 2   C = 2 gm/500 cc $\longrightarrow$ 2 $\underset{1\ 2\ 3}{000}$ mg/500 cc = **4 mg/cc**

   STEP 3 $\dfrac{DD}{C} = \dfrac{2\ \cancel{mg}/min}{4\ \cancel{mg}/cc}$ = **.5 cc/min**

4. STEP 1   DD = **25 mg**

   STEP 2   C = 50 mg/2 cc = **25 mg/cc**

   STEP 3 $\dfrac{DD}{C} = \dfrac{25\ \cancel{mg}}{25\ \cancel{mg}/cc}$ = **1 cc**

5. STEP 1   DD = 2 µg/kg/min ⟶ $2.2\overline{)2200}$ $\overset{100\,\textbf{kg}}{}$

                  ⟶ 100 × 2 µg = 200 µg

                    DD = **200 µg/min**

     STEP 2   C = 400 mg/500 cc = .8 mg/cc

               ⟶ .8 mg ⟶ 8 0 0. µg = **800 µg/cc**

     STEP 3 $\dfrac{DD}{C} = \dfrac{200\ \text{µg/min}}{800\ \text{µg/cc}} = $ **.25 cc/min**

6. STEP 1   DD = 1 mg/kg ⟶ $2.2\overline{)220}$ $\overset{10\,\textbf{kg}}{}$ ⟶ 10 × 1 mg = **10 mg**

     STEP 2   C = 100 mg/5 ml = **20 mg/ml**

     STEP 3 $\dfrac{DD}{C} = \dfrac{10\ \text{mg}}{20\ \text{mg/ml}} = $ **.5 ml**

7. STEP 1   DD = **12 mg**

     STEP 2   C = 20 mg/5 cc = **4 mg/cc**

     STEP 3 $\dfrac{DD}{C} = \dfrac{12\ \text{mg}}{4\ \text{mg/cc}} = $ **3 cc**

8. STEP 1   DD = **6 mg**

     STEP 2   C = 6 mg/2 cc = **3 mg/cc**

     STEP 3 $\dfrac{DD}{C} = \dfrac{6\ \text{mg}}{3\ \text{mg/cc}} = $ **2 cc**

9. STEP 1   DD = 8 µg/kg/min ⟶ $2.2\overline{)1450}$ $\overset{65.9\ \longrightarrow\ 66\,\textbf{kg}}{}$

                  ⟶ 66 × 8 µg = 528 µg

                    DD = **528 µg/min**

     STEP 2   C = 400 mg/250 cc = 1.6 mg/cc

               ⟶ 1.6 mg ⟶ 1 6 0 0. µg = **1600 µg/cc**

     STEP 3 $\dfrac{DD}{C} = \dfrac{528\ \text{µg/min}}{1600\ \text{µg/cc}} = $ **.33 cc/min**

10. STEP 1   DD = **3 mg/min**

     STEP 2   C = 1 gm/250 cc ⟶ 1 0 0 0 mg/250 cc = **4 mg/cc**

     STEP 3 $\dfrac{DD}{C} = \dfrac{3\ \text{mg/min}}{4\ \text{mg/cc}} = $ **.75 cc/min**

Chapter 4

Calculating Drip Rates

MIXING THE DRUG

To properly mix a drug **drip,** such as a Lidocaine drip, first determine the amount of the drug (in **cc's**) to be injected into the bag. **Then,** withdraw the equivalent amount of solution from the IV bag **prior** to mixing the drip. For example, Lidocaine comes supplied in a vial of 1 gm/**25 cc.** Therefore, since you will draw 25 cc from the vial and ultimately inject 25 cc of that drug into the IV bag, you must **first** draw 25 cc of fluid from the **bag.** So, after mixing the drip, you will have the **same** amount of **cc's** in the bag that you originally started with and that was used in the calculation of the concentration, e.g. 250 cc or 500 cc.

Failure to withdraw the equivalent amount of cc's from the bag **prior** to injecting the drug would alter the concentration that was originally calculated, thereby slightly affecting the **mg/min** being delivered. For example, if you were using a **250 cc** bag of normal saline and this being the figure that you used in your calculation, your **concentration** would actually be **weaker** because you would actually have **275 cc** in the bag after injecting the 25 cc of Lidocaine from the vial. This is only a point of concern, because too many times this information is not taught. In most cases this point of mention is of no grave consequence, but merely an issue of knowledge. However, when rendering care to the pediatric patient, this may be a concern to be reckoned with when administering sensitive medication to the small child, infant on neonat. Many times, especially in the emergency care field, there are premixed bags with such drugs as Lidocaine, dopamine, and many others. Premixed bags eliminate the need to withdraw fluid from the container prior to mixing. Generally, there are no further drug additives to be mixed into these pre-prepared drips in the prehospital world.

In reference to **gtt/cc,** this connotation indicates how many drops a particular administration set (or IV tubing) will deliver to produce 1 cc. In the health care field, there are generally two types of tubing. There are macrodrips and minidrips. Macrodrips are traditionally either 10 gtt/cc or 15 gtt/cc sets. These sets are used primarily to deliver a large volume of fluid over a short period of time. Minidrips are traditionally either 45 gtt/cc or 60 gtt/cc sets. These sets are used primarily to limit fluid intake and to administer medication intravenously. When dealing with drug drips in the field, the most common tubing is the minidrip administration set, which usually will deliver 60 drops per cc. Since the material in this guide is not geared toward traumatically injured patients, most scenarios will reflect nontraumatic emergency situations requiring minidrip sets, which will deliver 60 drops per cc.

Now that the following points have been clarified and the first three steps of this formula have been learned, we can proceed to the last and final step.

STEP 4

Calculate the **drip rate.** Calculating the rate is required to **deliver** the desired dose. The formula is:

$$\frac{cc \times gtt}{time}$$

In step 3, you recall that you calculated how many cc's were needed in order to administer the desired dose. To calculate step 4, **first** take the amount of **cc's** figured in step 3 and **multiply** that by the drip factor delivered by the administration set, which is **60** for a 60 gtt/cc set. See examples:

> 1 **cc** $\times$ 60 **gtt** = 60 gtt
>
> .213 **cc** $\times$ 60 **gtt** = 12.7 $\longrightarrow$ 13 gtt

After calculating the **cc** $\times$ 60 **gtt,** the **next** step is to **divide** the calculated drops (gtt) by the **time factor** found in the desired dose, which is normally 1 minute. See examples:

> $$\frac{1\,cc \times 60\,gtt}{\textbf{min}} = 60\ gtt/\textbf{min}$$
>
> $$\frac{.213\,cc \times 60\,gtt}{\textbf{min}} = 12.7 \longrightarrow 13\ gtt/\textbf{min}$$

If for some reason the doctor orders you to give so many cc/**hr,** which is common in both the clinical setting as well as in lengthy transports, you would need to break the **hour**(s) down into **minutes** and divide the total minutes into the calculation drops. See example:

$$\frac{150 \text{ cc} \times 60 \text{ gtt}}{1 \text{ hr} \,(\mathbf{60\ min})} = \frac{9000 \text{ gtt}}{\mathbf{60\ min}} = 150 \text{ gtt/min}$$

Notice that after multiplying **cc × gtt,** you automatically eliminate the **measurement** of cc's, with an end result of drops per minute. Don't neglect to remember the rule of **canceling** out numbers. In the above example, to simplify this equation, you can cancel out 60 in both the numerator and the denominator. See example:

$$\frac{150 \text{ cc} \times \cancel{60} \text{ gtt}}{\cancel{60} \text{ min}} = 150 \text{ gtt/min}$$

A note especially for those professionals in the clinical setting: many times a physician will give an order for so many **cc's** an **hour** to be given. With this information, step **3** has been calculated for you by the physician. Many times when a doctor orders so many cc/hr, he or she also instructs you how to mix the drip especially in the clinical setting. So, in essence, the only calculation that you have to deal with is **step 4** (calculating the drip rate). But, we must be mindful that even though this information may be provided by a licensed physician, it remains the caregiver's responsibility to ensure that the proper dosage ordered is being delivered.

In recent years, examiners have included on some of their tests what they refer to as a backward dopamine drip. The following is an example of this problem.

You have been ordered to initiate a **dopamine drip.** Your on-hand concentration is **1600 μg/cc.** The patient's weight is **150** pounds, and you are using a minidrip tubing that delivers **60 gtt/cc.** Your patient is receiving **8 gtt/min.** How many μg/kg is your patient receiving?

a. 3 μg/kg
b. 4 μg/kg
c. 5 μg/kg
d. 6 μg/kg

People tend to assume that this question is very complex. However, it is extremely simple. By now, you should have the basic concepts of the formula memorized. All of the information that you need to figure this problem has been given. One way to calculate the correct answer is to work the problem out using each answer (a, b, c, & d) until your answer matches the drops per minute that your patient is receiving, which is given to you in the problem. In the following example, you will discover, that answer **(a) 3 mg/kg** will render **8 gtt/min** as stated in the question.

Answer: **(a) 3 μg/kg**

STEP 1   DD = **3 μg/kg**/min ⟶ $2.2\overline{)1500}$ 68 **kg**

⟶ 68 × 3 μg = 204 μg

$$\text{DD} = 204 \ \mu g/min$$

STEP 2 $\text{C} = 1600 \ \mu g/cc$ (given in the question)

STEP 3 $\dfrac{\text{DD}}{\text{C}} = \dfrac{204 \ \mu g/min}{1600 \ \mu g/cc} = .127 \ cc/min$

STEP 4 $\dfrac{\mathbf{cc \times gtt}}{\mathbf{time}} = \dfrac{.127 \ cc \times 60 \ gtt}{min} = 7.6 \ \mathbf{gtt} \longrightarrow \mathbf{8 \ gtt/min}$

Following are some practice questions showing the calculations for this step.

An order has been given for a dopamine **drip** to be run at **200 mg/min.** Your concentration is **1600 μg/cc**. How many gtt/min must you deliver using a **60 gtt** administration set?

STEP 1 $\text{DD} = 200 \ \mu g/min$

STEP 2 $\text{C} = 1600 \ \mu g/cc$

STEP 3 $\dfrac{\text{DD}}{\text{C}} = \dfrac{200 \ \mu g/min}{1600 \ \mu g/cc} = .125 \ cc/min$

STEP 4 $\dfrac{\mathbf{cc \times gtt}}{\mathbf{time}} = \dfrac{.125 \ cc \times 60 \ gtt}{min} = 7.5 \ gtt \longrightarrow \mathbf{8 \ gtt/min}$

An order has been given for **2 mg/min** via Lidocaine **drip**. Your concentration is **4 mg/cc**. How many gtt/min would you deliver using a **minidrip**?

STEP 1 $\text{DD} = 2 \ mg/min$

STEP 2 $\text{C} = 4 \ mg/cc$

STEP 3 $\dfrac{\text{DD}}{\text{C}} = \dfrac{2 \ mg/min}{4 \ mg/cc} = .5 \ cc/min$

STEP 4 $\dfrac{\mathbf{cc \times gtt}}{\mathbf{time}} = \dfrac{.5 \ cc \times 60 \ gtt}{min} = \mathbf{30 \ gtt/min}$

An order has been given for a particular premixed bag of theophylline to be run at **150 cc/hr** using a **minidrip.** How many gtt/min would you deliver?

STEP 1 $\text{DD} = skip$

STEP 2 $\text{C} = skip$

STEP 3 $\dfrac{\text{DD}}{\text{C}} = skip$

STEP 4 $\dfrac{\mathbf{cc \times gtt}}{\mathbf{time}} = \dfrac{150 \ cc \times 60 \ gtt}{(1 \ hr) \ 60 \ min} = \mathbf{150 \ gtt/min}$

As you noticed, the concentration was **not** given in this problem. Remember, the concentration was not necessary to calculate the gtt/min, because the doctor has ordered you to use a particular premixed bag and had already given you the **cc/hr** to give. So the only step that you have to deal with in this particular problem is **step 4,** on calculating the **gtt/min.**

An order has been given for **20 mg/min** of **procainamide** via IV **drip.** Your concentration is **20 mg/cc.** How many gtt/min would you deliver using a **60 gtt** set?

STEP 1   DD = 20 mg/min

STEP 2   C = 20 mg/cc

STEP 3 $\dfrac{DD}{C} = \dfrac{20 \text{ mg/min}}{20 \text{ mg/cc}} = 1 \text{ cc/min}$

STEP 4 $\dfrac{\textbf{cc} \times \textbf{gtt}}{\textbf{time}} = \dfrac{\textbf{1 cc} \times \textbf{60 gtt}}{\textbf{min}} = \textbf{60 gtt/min}$

In the above example, after calculating step **3,** your answer was **1 cc/min.** By looking at this answer, you know that the drops per minute will be 60 without multiplying 1 cc × 60 gtt, because you know that with a minidrip, the drip factor is 60 gtt/**cc.** So, if you want to give 1 cc per min, this would take 60 gtt.

An order has been given for **10 μg/min** of a given drug via drip. Your concentration is **4 μg/cc.** How many gtt/min would you deliver using a **minidrip**?

STEP 1   DD = 10 μg/min

STEP 2   C = 4 μg/cc

STEP 3 $\dfrac{DD}{C} = \dfrac{10 \text{ μg/min}}{4 \text{ μg/cc}} = 2.5 \text{ cc/min}$

STEP 4 $\dfrac{\textbf{cc} \times \textbf{gtt}}{\textbf{time}} = \dfrac{\textbf{2.5 cc} \times \textbf{60 gtt}}{\textbf{min}} = \textbf{150 gtt/min}$

SUMMARY

Always be **consistent** in following each step, whether you are calculating **cc's** to draw or calculating **drips.** Now you have learned the **easy, 4-step method to drug calculations:**

STEP 1   **DD**

STEP 2   **C (always weight/cc)**
           e.g.—mg/cc

STEP 3 $\dfrac{\textbf{DD}}{\textbf{C}}$

STEP 4 $\dfrac{\textbf{cc} \times \textbf{gtt}}{\textbf{time}}$

Congratulations! Good luck on your class and state exams.

Review

Now that you know how to calculate all four steps of this formula, following are some practice questions requiring you to calculate some drip rates:

1. You have been ordered to initiate a **Lidocaine drip** using a premixed bag. You are to give **3 mg/min.** Your concentration is **4 mg/cc,** and you're using a **60 gtt/cc** set. How many **drops per minute** must you deliver?

2. You have been ordered to initiate a **dopamine drip** to be run at 2 µg/kg/min. After calculating the patient's weight, you will be giving **200 µg/min.** Your concentration is **800 µg/cc.** You will be giving **.25 cc/min** using a **minidrip** administration set. How many gtt/min must you deliver?

3. You have been ordered to deliver **200 cc/hr** of a premixed **amino-phylline drip** for the first hour. **After** the **first** hour, the doctor wants you to deliver the remainder at **125 cc/hr.** Using a **minidrip,** what is your **gtt/min** for the remaining aminophylline?

4. You have been ordered to initiate a **procainamide drip** to be run at **20 mg/min**. On hand is a vial containing **1 gm,** a **50 cc** bag, and a **minidrip** tubing. How many **drops per minute** would you deliver with a patient weight of **225** pounds?

5. You have received orders to start a **Nipride drip** to be run at **.5 μg/kg/min.** On hand you have **50 mg** of **Nipride,** a **250 ml** container, and a **minidrip.** The patient's weight is **154** pounds. How many **drops per minute** would you deliver?

6. A **dopamine drip** has been ordered to be run at **2 μg/kg/min.** On hand, you have a **400 mg** vial, a **500 cc** bag of normal saline, and a **60 gtt/cc** administration set. Your patient's weight is **188** pounds. How many **drops per minute** would you deliver?

7. You have been ordered to start a maintenance **infusion** of **aminophylline** to be run at **.5 mg/kg/hr.** Your patient weighs **202** pounds. On hand you have a **250 cc** bag of normal saline, **two** vials, containing **250 mg** in each, and a **minidrip**. How many **drops per minute** would you deliver?

8. You have been ordered to give **.5 mg/kg** of **Lidocaine** IVP, followed by a **Lidocaine drip** to be run at **2 mg/min.** On hand you have a **5 cc** prefilled syringe containing **100 mg**, **two** vials containing **1 gm** in **each**, a **500 cc** bag of normal saline, and a **minidrip.** Your patient weighs **175** pounds.
    a. Using the prefilled syringe, how many **cc's** would you give IVP?

    b. How many **drops per minute** would you deliver via IV **drip**?

9. You have a patient scheduled for surgery for whom the doctor has ordered an **Ancef drip** running a **50 cc** bag of normal saline over a **30-minute** time frame. On hand is a minidrip and a vial containing **1 gm** of **Ancef,** which is supplied in powder form into which you will dilute 2 cc of fluid. How many **drops per minute** would you deliver to give the **desired dose**?

10. You have been ordered to initiate a **dopamine drip** to be run at **5 μg/kg/min.** On hand are **two** vials containing **200 mg** in **each,** a **250 cc** bag of normal saline, and a **60 gtt** set. Your patient weights **143** pounds. How many **drops per minute** would you deliver?

Answers

1. STEP 1 DD = **3 mg/min**

   STEP 2 C = **4 mg/cc**

   STEP 3 $\dfrac{DD}{C} = \dfrac{3\ \text{mg/min}}{4\ \text{mg/cc}} = $ **.75 cc/min**

   STEP 4 $\dfrac{\text{cc} \times \text{gtt}}{\text{time}} = \dfrac{.75\ \text{cc} \times 60\ \text{gtt}}{\text{min}} = $ **45 gtt/min**

2. STEP 1 DD = **200 μg/min**

   STEP 2 C = **800 μg/cc**

   STEP 3 $\dfrac{DD}{C} = \dfrac{200\ \text{μg/min}}{800\ \text{μg/cc}} = $ **.25 cc/min**

   STEP 4 $\dfrac{\text{cc} \times \text{gtt}}{\text{time}} = \dfrac{.25\ \text{cc} \times 60\ \text{gtt}}{\text{min}} = $ **15 gtt/min**

3. STEP 1 DD = Skip

   STEP 2 C = Skip

   STEP 3 $\dfrac{DD}{C} = $ Skip

STEP 4 $\dfrac{cc \times gtt}{time} = \dfrac{125 \text{ cc} \times \cancel{60} \text{ gtt}}{\cancel{60} \text{ min}} = \mathbf{125 \text{ gtt/min}}$

4. STEP 1 DD = **20 mg/min**

   STEP 2 C = 1 gm/50 cc $\longrightarrow$ 1 0 0 0 mg/50 cc = **20 mg/cc**

   STEP 3 $\dfrac{DD}{C} = \dfrac{20 \cancel{\text{ mg}}/min}{20 \cancel{\text{ mg}}/cc} = \mathbf{1 \text{ cc/min}}$

   STEP 4 $\dfrac{cc \times gtt}{time} = \dfrac{1 \text{ cc} \times 60 \text{ gtt}}{min} = \mathbf{60 \text{ gtt/min}}$

5. STEP 1 DD = .5 μg/kg/min $\longrightarrow$ $2.2 \overline{\smash{)}1540}$ 70 kg

   $\longrightarrow 70 \times .5 \text{ μg} = 35 \text{ μg}$

   DD = **35 μg/min**

   STEP 2 C = 50 mg/250 ml = .2 mg/ml

   $\longrightarrow .2 \text{ mg} \longrightarrow 2 0 0. \text{ μg} = \mathbf{200 \text{ μg/ml}}$

   STEP 3 $\dfrac{DD}{C} = \dfrac{35 \cancel{\text{ μg}}/min}{200 \cancel{\text{ μg}}/ml} = \mathbf{.175 \text{ ml/min}}$

   STEP 4 $\dfrac{cc \times gtt}{time} = \dfrac{.175 \text{ ml} \times 60 \text{ gtt}}{min} = 10.5 \longrightarrow \mathbf{11 \text{ gtt/min}}$

6. STEP 1 DD = 2 μg/kg/min $\longrightarrow$ $2.2 \overline{\smash{)}1880}$ 85.45 $\longrightarrow$ 86 kg

   $\longrightarrow 86 \times 2 \text{ μg} = 172 \text{ μg}$

   DD = **172 μg/min**

   STEP 2 C = 400 mg/500 cc = .8 mg/cc

   $\longrightarrow .8 \text{ mg} \longrightarrow 8 0 0. \text{ μg} = \mathbf{800 \text{ μg/cc}}$

   STEP 3 $\dfrac{DD}{C} = \dfrac{172 \cancel{\text{ μg}}/min}{800 \cancel{\text{ μg}}/cc} = \mathbf{.215 \text{ cc/min}}$

   STEP 4 $\dfrac{cc \times gtt}{time} = \dfrac{.215 \text{ cc} \times 60 \text{ gtt}}{min} = 12.9 \longrightarrow \mathbf{13 \text{ gtt/min}}$

7. STEP 1 DD = .5 mg/kg/hr $\longrightarrow$ $2.2 \overline{\smash{)}2020}$ 91.8 $\longrightarrow$ 92 kg

   $\longrightarrow 92 \times .5 \text{ mg} = 46 \text{ mg}$

   DD = **46 mg/hr**

   STEP 2 C = 500 mg/250 cc = **2 mg/cc**

   STEP 3 $\dfrac{DD}{C} = \dfrac{46 \cancel{\text{ mg}}/hr}{2 \cancel{\text{ mg}}/cc} = \mathbf{23 \text{ cc/hr}}$

   STEP 4 $\dfrac{cc \times gtt}{time} = \dfrac{23 \text{ cc} \times \cancel{60} \text{ gtt}}{\cancel{60} \text{ min (1 hr)}} = \mathbf{23 \text{ gtt/min}}$

8. a. STEP 1   DD = .5 mg/kg $\longrightarrow$ $2.2\overline{)1750}$ $\xrightarrow{79.5}$ 80 kg

                           $\longrightarrow$ 80 × .5 mg = **40 mg**

                                 DD = 40 mg

         STEP 2   C = 100 mg/5 cc = **20 mg/cc**

         STEP 3 $\dfrac{DD}{C} = \dfrac{40 \text{ mg}}{20 \text{ mg/cc}} = \textbf{2 cc}$

     b. STEP 1   DD = **2 mg/min**

         STEP 2   C = 2 gm/500 cc $\longrightarrow$ $2\underset{1\ 2\ 3}{\underbrace{0\ 0\ 0}}$ mg/500 cc = **4 mg/cc**

         STEP 3 $\dfrac{DD}{C} = \dfrac{2 \text{ mg/min}}{4 \text{ mg/cc}} = \textbf{.5 cc/min}$

         STEP 4 $\dfrac{cc \times gtt}{time} = \dfrac{.5 \text{ cc} \times 60 \text{ gtt}}{min} = \textbf{30 gtt/min}$

9. STEP 1   DD = Skip

     STEP 2   C = Skip

     STEP 3 $\dfrac{DD}{C}$ = Skip

     STEP 4 $\dfrac{cc \times gtt}{time} = \dfrac{50 \text{ cc} \times 60 \text{ gtt}}{30 \text{ min}} = \textbf{100 gtt/min}$

10. STEP 1   DD = 5 μg/kg/min $\longrightarrow$ $2.2\overline{)1430}$ $\xrightarrow{65 \text{ kg}}$

                              $\longrightarrow$ 65 × 5 μg = 325 μg

                           DD = 325 μg/min

      STEP 2   C = 400 mg/250 cc = **1.6 mg/cc**

                  $\longrightarrow$ 1.6 mg $\longrightarrow$ $1\underset{1\ 2\ 3}{\underbrace{6\ 0\ 0}}.$ μg = **1600 μg/cc**

      STEP 3 $\dfrac{DD}{C} = \dfrac{325 \text{ μg/min}}{1600 \text{ μg/cc}} = \textbf{.203 cc/min}$

      STEP 4 $\dfrac{cc \times gtt}{time} = \dfrac{.203 \text{ cc} \times 60 \text{ gtt}}{min} = 12.1 \longrightarrow \textbf{12 gtt/min}$

Final Review

1. Most of your patients in an air ambulance are in critical condition. You have received a call to a baseball field in a small town about **45** minutes away by air. When you arrive, your 17-year-old patient has been packaged by the local EMS. They advise you that the patient was struck in the **head** by a baseball bat about an hour ago and **lost** consciousness. His initial vital signs were P–**90,** BP–**120/80,** R–**18,** and his condition has continued to deteriorate rapidly. Upon further evaluation, you find that the patient's left **pupil** is **blown** (i.e., fixed and dilated), and he is **unconscious** and **unresponsive,** with **projectile vomiting.** His vital signs are P–**54,** BP–**162/94,** R–**24** and **erratic.** An IV has been established; however, there has been no drug intervention. You are now en route to the medical center awaiting further orders from the ED. The ED physician on duty contacts you by radio and orders you to administer **4 mg** of **Decadron** IVP. On hand is a **5 ml** vial containing **20 mg.** How many ml's will you give?

2. You've just finished your afternoon coffee break at the Hurricane Surfer, which is the most popular coffee shop on the beach, when you are dispatched to the ship docks for a possible **overdose.** A police officer on scene advises you that the scene is secure and that your patient is a known habitual **heroin** abuser. Upon arrival, you find your patient to be in a **comatose** state, his pupils **constricted,** and he is experiencing **respiratory depression.** While your partner is securing the airway and assisting the breathing via BVM, you discover **tracks** on both arms. You are unable to find a good vein in which to establish an IV, so you decide to administer **2 mg** of **Narcan** IM. On hand, you have a **10 cc** vial containing **4 mg** of **Narcan.** How many cc's must you draw in order to deliver the desired dose?

3. You have been dispatched to Park Crest Manor for a 74-year-old female complaining of **difficulty** breathing. When you arrive, your patient is sitting on the edge of the bed experiencing severe **dyspnea** with **cyanosis** evident in her nail beds and sclera. Upon further examination, you also find that she has a **history** of **congestive heart failure.** Upon auscultation of the lungs, you note **basilar rales** and notice that she is using her accessory muscles to further assist her breathing. You recognize that her dyspnea is most likely secondary to the **pulmonary edema** that is present. While your partner is giving oxygen, you have established an IV and have decided to administer **40 mg** of **Lasix** IVP. On hand is a **4 ml** prefilled syringe containing **40 mg.** How many ml's will you need to push?

4. It's lunch time and you're on the way to the Pizza Palace when your pager goes off, dispatching you to Gazebo Courts Nursing Home for a patient experiencing an **altered state of consciousness.** The nurse states that this is a new resident who has been extremely **agitated** for the past day or so. Upon evaluation, you find the patient is having **trouble** speaking and is complaining of **tightness** in his **jaw** and of a **stiff neck.** You also notice that his head appears to be **deviated** to the left. When you inquire as to what medications this patient is taking, the nurse states that he is on **Haldol** PRN and that he has taken at least **six times** his normal dosage. After relaying this information to medical control, they order you to give **50 mg** of **Benadryl** IV in an attempt to reverse the patient's **extrapyramidal reaction.** On hand is a **2 cc** vial containing **50 mg** of Benadryl. How many cc's must you give?

5. Today, your partner is a new hire who just received his paramedic certification. When you are dispatched to a 70-year-old female who has **passed out,** he beats you to the ambulance. When you arrive, you have to remind your partner to calm down. When you enter the residence, your patient is lying in bed, **conscious,** and complaining of mild **chest pain** and **palpitations** in her chest. When you hook up the monitor, you see that your patient is in **PSVT** with an HR of **170.** All other vitals are **stable.** At that time, you're thinking that this would be a great opportunity for your new partner to actually get to do something. The patient advises you that she has a history of **PSVT** and **carotid artery disease.** She also states that she is **allergic** to **adenosine** and that she does **not** have **Wolff–Parkinson–White syndrome.** After giving oxygen and establishing an IV, you decide to let your partner give a dose of **verapamil.** While your partner is tending to the **verapamil** administration, you get involved in communicating with the patient. **Ten** minutes into the transport, the patient begins to complain of feeling extremely **weak** and **passes out,** at which time you take her blood pressure. The best pressure you can get is **40/P.** You knew that **verapamil** could cause some **hypotension,** but you didn't expect it to be this severe. You then ask your new partner how much **verapamil** he gave her, and he tells you 10 mg. Now you know why the patient is so hypotensive; it's because too much was given initially. You immediately decide to give **.5 gm** of **calcium chloride** in an attempt to reverse this untoward effect. On hand is a **10 cc** prefilled syringe containing **1 gm.** How many cc's will you administer?

6. While you are relaxing at the EMS station, a frantic mother runs in and states that her 2-year-old son is having a difficult time **breathing.** You find the child to be experiencing a severe **asthma attack** with **wheezing** in all fields. It becomes necessary to give **.01 mg/kg** of **epinephrine 1:1000** sq. On hand, you have an ampule containing **1 mg** in **1 cc.** The mother advises you that her son weighs approximately **22** pounds. How many cc's will you give?

7. "We finally made it back to the station at 4:00 this morning. At least we can get a few hours of sleep before we head home." But at 6:00 a.m. the pager goes off, dispatching you on a medical emergency. You arrive on scene to find a 54-year-old male in **respiratory distress.** The patient advises you that he has **lost** quite a bit of **weight** lately and that it seems like his **shortness of breath** has been getting worse. While your patient is coughing, you notice a large ashtray on the night stand overflowing with cigarette butts. The patient states that he has been smoking two packs a day for 20 years. During your physical exam, you notice that the patient appears to be **pink** in color, **thin,** and somewhat **barrel chested.** It is obvious that this patient is a **"pink puffer"** and is suffering from **emphysema.** After giving an Albuterol breathing treatment, your patient becomes **unresponsive** and **apneic.** When you look at the EKG monitor, you notice that your patient is **bradycardic** with a HR of **34.** Immediately following intubation, you decide to administer **atropine.** With IV access **not** readily available, you decide to give **atropine** via an **ET tube.** Your normal dose would be **.5 mg,** but knowing that the dosage needs to be **doubled,** you decide to give **1 mg** ET. On hand is a **10 cc** prefilled syringe containing **1 mg.** How many cc's must you give?

8. You have a 59-year-old female complaining of **weakness** and **chest pain.** She states that she has **heart disease** and that she had an **MI** two years ago. She also states that for the past few hours it feels like her heart has been **"skipping beats."** The cardiac monitor shows a sinus rhythm with **bigeminy PVCs** and occasional **couplets.** After administering oxygen, according to protocol, you must administer **1 mg/kg** of **Lidocaine** IVP. Your patient's weight is **140 pounds.** On hand is a **5 ml** prefilled syringe containing **100 mg** of **Lidocaine.** How many ml's must you deliver?

9. You've received a call to a retirement home for a 78-year-old female having **difficulty breathing.** When you arrive, you find that the patient is very **weak, cool,** and somewhat **diaphoretic.** Upon further evaluation, you discover **audible rales** in all lobes as well as **pedal edema.** Your patient's BP is **98/P** and she weighs close to **200** pounds. She states that her past medical history consists of CHF and pneumonia. After giving a dose of Lasix, you decide to go ahead with a **dobutamine drip** run at **2.5 µg/kg/min.** On hand is a **250 mg** vial, a **500 cc** bag of fluid, and a **minidrip** administration set. How many gtt/min must you deliver?

10. It's time for the Firemen's Annual Chili Cookoff. While you're sitting around enjoying a bowl of chili, the fire chief comes to you and says that a child was stung by a bee while playing underneath a picnic table. He wants you to go over and check out the little 4-year-old boy. Upon arrival, the mother states that he is **allergic** to **bees** and that he has a **history** of asthma, which can make matters worse. Upon evaluation, you find **hives** on his **hands, arms, neck,** and **face,** as well as some **wheezing** and **upper airway stridor.** You quickly recognize that this child is possibly going into **anaphylaxis** and that his condition is life threatening. While your partner is maintaining the airway and giving oxygen, you establish an IV of normal saline. The mother states that her son weighs around **40** pounds. Since you have determined that this patient needs to be treated for anaphylaxis, you have given .01 mg/kg of Epi 1:10,000. There now seems to be some relief, but you wish to follow up with **2 mg/kg** of **Benadryl** IV. On hand is a **1 cc** vial containing **50 mg.** How many cc's must you administer?

11. You have been dispatched to the scene of a pediatric overdose. Upon arrival, you find a 5-year-old child lying in the living room **unconscious** and **unresponsive.** The grandmother states that while they were reading books, she noticed that her grandson's **speech** sounded very slurred. However, at the time she didn't think much of it. About an hour later, her grandson **passed out.** When she went to the bathroom to get a wet rag, she noticed that he had gotten into the medicine cabinet. The only bottle that she found open was her **Elavil,** which is a **tricyclic antidepressant.** Upon further evaluation, you find that your patient's respiratory rate is **12,** both pupils are **dilated,** and that he is in **sinus tachycardia.** At this point, you suspect that your patient is suffering from a possible **tricyclic overdose.** While your partner maintains the airway, you establish IV access. According to protocol, you need to administer **1 mEq/kg** of **sodium bicarbonate.** You estimate that the child's weight is around **40** pounds. On hand is a **50 cc** prefilled syringe containing **50 mEq.** How many cc's will you administer to deliver the desired dose?

12. The Emergency Department is really hopping this evening, and you've just arrived with your sixth patient of the day. While cleaning out the back of your unit, a car pulls up to the ED entrance, and someone hollers for your help. When you get over to the car, you find a male in his **early 20s,** very **anxious** and complaining of **chest pain.** When you get your patient into the ED, the nurse asks you to evaluate him. After hooking up the monitor, you discover **SVT** with a sustained HR of **220.** Also, you note his **dilated** pupils, involuntary **twitching** of muscles, as well as a BP of **180/110.** You ask your patient if he has done any drugs recently. He advises you that he was at a party and that he freebased more **crack** than he normally does. It's obvious that this patient is suffering from a **crack cocaine overdose.** You report these findings to the ED physician. Knowing that **benzodiazepines** are generally the **first-line drugs** given to **cocaine overdose** patients, you were able to anticipate the physician's order. Subsequently, the ED physician orders you to give **5 mg** of **diazepam** IV. On hand is a **2 ml** vial containing **10 mg** of **Valium.** How many ml's must you draw?

13. A call comes in about a man down in the city park. You arrive at the scene to find your patient is covered with **erythema** (red rash), **urticaria** is present on both arms, and **facial edema** is observed. Within seconds, your patient becomes very **restless** and begins to experience **upper airway stridor.** It has been determined that your patient is experiencing a **severe allergic reaction,** which is quickly progressing toward **anaphylaxis.** While your partner maintains the patient's airway, you take a BP of **80/40** and establish an IV of normal saline. Protocol directs you to give **.5 mg** of **epinephrine 1:10,000,** slow IVP. On hand is a **10 ml** prefilled syringe with **1 mg.** How many ml's will you push?

14. A 911 call has come in about a man down in an alley. You know this area to be the local hangout for the homeless. When you arrive, everybody is sitting around drinking **wine** and **beer.** You notice your patient lying on the ground, **unconscious** and **unresponsive.** One bystander states that your patient is an **alcoholic** and that he has been having a lot of **stomach problems** lately. Another bystander states that your patient has **passed out** several times today, but this time he hasn't come around for a good 15 minutes or so. Upon further evaluation, you find your patient to be **diaphoretic** and **tachycardic.** While your partner gives oxygen and maintains the airway, you establish an IV of normal saline. Prior to giv-

ing D50, you must administer **100 mg** of **thiamine** IVP. On hand is a **1 cc** vial containing **100 mg.** How many cc's will you administer?

15. You have been dispatched on a 911 call to the far north end of the county, which is about 45 minutes away, for a man who has **passed out.** When you arrive, you find a 68-year-old male **conscious** sitting up in a chair, complaining of some **mild chest discomfort,** with a BP of **98/60.** The cardiac monitor is showing a **second-degree AV block,** which you recognize to be **Type I Wenckebach** with a HR of **70.** After placing your patient on the stretcher, he becomes extremely **weak** and his heart rate drops to **38 bpm.** Upon confirming that there has been no change in his respiratory status, you give oxygen, establish an IV of normal saline, and administer .5 mg of atropine. His HR has now increased to **58 bpm,** but his BP has dropped to **82/58.** You have given a 300 cc bolus of normal saline, which has not increased the BP. However, the patient's HR has now increased to a comfortable 70 bpm. Protocol states to initiate a **dopamine drip,** to be run at **5 mcg/kg/min,** after which you should titrate to the BP. Your patient states that he weighs about **280 pounds.** On hand is a **10 ml** vial containing **400 mg** of **dopamine,** a **250 cc** bag of normal saline, and a **60 gtt** administration set. How many gtt/min must you deliver?

16. You have been dispatched to 1000 Memory Lane for a 17-year-old male who has possibly **overdosed** on **Valium.** When you arrive on scene, the frantic mother advises you that her son must have gotten into her purse and taken her pill bottle, which was missing about **30** of her **Valium tablets.** She also states that her son has been extremely **depressed** over the death of his high school girlfriend. Upon evaluation, you find your patient **semiconscious, bradycardic,** and experiencing **respiratory depression.** The mother states that this was the only medication in her purse and that the pill bottle was open when she found it beside her son's bed. Since the Valium appears to have been the **only** drug that was ingested, according to protocol, you are to administer **.2 mg** of Flumazenil **(Romazicon)** IV. On hand is a **10 cc** vial containing **1 mg** of **Romazicon.** How many cc's must you give?

17. You have been called to the scene of a 36-year-old female complaining of a **severe headache.** Upon evaluating your patient, you find her to be 38 weeks **pregnant** with a BP of **200/116,** and **pedal edema** is present. She states that last week her physician discovered **protein** in her urine as well as **excessive weight gain.** You have determined that your patient is experiencing **pregnancy-induced hypertension** (PID). After contacting the ED with your patient report, they advise you that the patient will need a dose of **Apresoline** when you arrive at the ED. When you arrive at the busy emergency room, your medical director, who happens to be the ED physician, orders you to administer **10 mg** of **Apresoline** IV. On hand is a **2 cc** ampule containing **20 mg.** How many cc's will you give?

18. You have been dispatched to the bus station downtown for an obstetrical emergency. Upon arrival, you find a 26-year-old female in her **second trimester** of **pregnancy.** Your patient advises you that shortly after arriving at the station, she became **weak** and began seeing **spots** and **flashing lights.** Upon evaluation, you find a BP of **180/110** as well as marked **edema.** At this point, you are assuming that your patient may be suffering from possible **pre-eclampsia.** After administering oxygen and establishing a line of normal saline, Medical Control orders you to give **1 gm** of **magnesium sulfate** IVP. On hand, you have a **10 cc** prefilled syringe with **5 gm** of **magnesium sulfate.** How many cc's must you administer in order to give your desired dose?

19. While you are working in the ED as a paramedic, EMS brings in a **post-CPR** patient who has successfully been revived following aggressive V-fib protocol. It has been about 10 minutes since the cardiac arrest, and the patient's BP is **70/30.** The ED physician orders you to initiate a **dopamine drip** to be run at **6 μg/kg/min.** The patient's estimated weight is **200** pounds. On hand is a vial containing **400 mg** of **dopamine,** a **250 cc** bag of normal saline, and a **minidrip** administration set. At what flow rate would you run the dopamine drip?

20. It's a hot summer day, and the lake is busy. You have been dispatched to a man injured in a **diving accident.** When you arrive, you find a by-stander kneeling on the ground holding the patient's C-spine. This 19-year-old patient states that he dove out of the boat into what he believed to be deep water, but in fact was only three feet of water. His friends state that he was **"knocked out"** for a few minutes. The patient's only complaint is **severe neck pain.** Upon further evaluation, you find a **loss of sensation** below the **nipple line, paralysis,** and **priapism.** The patient's C-spine is immobilized, vitals are stable, oxygen is being given, and you have an IV established. You have determined that your patient most likely has a **spinal cord injury** somewhere in the thoracic spine. For spinal cord injuries, protocol states that you must administer **30 mg/kg** of **Solumedrol** over a **15-minute** period. On hand is a vial containing **2000 mg** of **Solumedrol** in powder form, which you have diluted with 5 cc of fluid, a **50 cc** bag of normal saline, and a **60 gtt** administration set. Your patient's weight is **132** pounds.

a. How many cc's must you draw from the vial to be mixed in the drip?

b. How many drops per minute would you deliver?

21. One of your routine patients, Mr. Green, is complaining of a sudden on-set of **weakness.** From past experience, you know that he has an extensive cardiac history. You attach the cardiac monitor to find that Mr. Green is in **third-degree heart block** with a HR of **42 bpm.** He has a BP of **92/64,** which is **hypotensive** for this six-foot, 200-pound man. Medical Control has ordered you to perform transcutaneous cardiac pacing (TCP). As you are loading Mr. Green into the ambulance, he starts to complain about some **discomfort** in his **chest.** After further evaluation, you determine that his discomfort is most likely coming from the pac-ing, which occasionally happens in these patients. Since his vital signs have improved, with a BP of **112/68** and a HR of **72,** you have received verbal orders via telephone from the ED physician to administer **2 mg**

of **versed** (midazolam) IV in an attempt to relieve the patient's discomfort. On hand is a **2 ml** vial containing **10 mg** of **midazolam.** How many ml's must you administer to deliver the desired dose?

22. Never say "I hope we have a slow day today," because it will always backfire on you. It's Saturday afternoon, and your station is toned out to a child **seizing.** When you arrive, the father is outside the garage rinsing his son off with the water hose. The father states that while he was mowing the yard, his 3-year-old son got into the **insecticides.** When he found him, his son was covered in **insecticide dust** and **granules** and appeared to be **seizing.** Upon further evaluation, you find the boy to be responsive only to **deep stimuli.** He is **vomiting,** has **constricted pupils,** and **excessive salivation,** but at present has no seizure activity. Now that the boy's clothes have been removed and the insecticide has been rinsed off, you determine that this child is suffering from **organophosphate poisoning.** While your partner is taking care of the child's airway, you establish an IV. According to protocol, you must start with **.05 mg/kg** of **atropine** IVP in an attempt to **dry up** the secretions. The father states that his son weighs **38** pounds. On hand is a **20 ml** vial containing **8 mg** of **atropine.** How many ml's will you give?

23. You are called to the residence of a 65-year-old male complaining of **weakness.** Upon evaluation, you discover that your patient is **hypotensive** with a BP of **70/40.** The patient states that he experienced a **syncopal episode** earlier this morning. The cardiac monitor is showing **third-degree heart block** with a HR of **40.** Since transcutaneous cardiac pacing is **not** available, you must administer **.5** mg of atropine. It has been 10 minutes, and the HR is now up to **72 bpm;** however, your patient's blood pressure has **not** improved. You have decided to initiate a **dopamine drip** to be run at **2 μg/kg/min.** Your patient's weight is **180** pounds. On hand is a vial containing **200 mg** of **dopamine,** a **250 cc** bag of normal saline, and a **minidrip** set. How many drops per minute must you deliver?

24. You received a call to a construction site for a man experiencing **chest pain.** Upon arrival, you find a 45-year-old male sitting on the ground, **conscious** and **alert** × 3, **short of breath,** and **diaphoretic.** While your partner is hooking up the oxygen, you apply the cardiac monitor. You find a sinus rhythm with frequent unifocal **PVCs** that occasionally fall **almost** on the **T-wave.** While initiating an IV of normal saline, your patient quickly deteriorates into **V-tach** and immediately into pulseless **V-fib.** After delivering three shocks at 200, 300, and 360, your patient converts into a sinus rhythm with an HR of **80,** with a depressed ST segment and a good strong palpable pulse. According to protocol, you must give a 1.5 mg/kg bolus of **Lidocaine.** Now you need to follow up with a **Lidocaine drip** as a **prophylactic** against **recurrent V-fib.** On hand is a vial containing **1 gm** of **Lidocaine,** a **250 cc** bag of solution, and a **minidrip** administration set. According to protocol, you must run the drip at **4 mg/min.** How many gtt/min must you deliver?

25. "Put your coat back on; we're going on another call." You've been dispatched to Jennifer's Miracle Workout and Exercise Club for a 42-year-old man having an **asthma attack.** On the way to the scene, you have a flashback and recall the first asthmatic call you ever responded to. You met that patient on a country road on his way to the hospital. You recall how that patient became a statistic of the many patients who die each year from asthma. You say to yourself, "Well, that's not going to happen with this patient." When you arrive on the scene, you find your patient to be very **anxious** and **agitated.** Your assessment reveals **severe difficulty** breathing, **wheezing, coughing, speech dyspnea,** and **tachycardia.** Your patient states that he had just finished exercising and that the **cold** outside must have **triggered** his attack. Also, the last time this happened he had to be **intubated** and **ventilated.** You've only been on scene for a minute or two, and your patient acts as if he is ready to **pass out.** Oxygen sats are **84%,** respirations are **28,** HR is **130,** and BP is **144/92.** You administer high-flow oxygen while your partner is preparing a neb treatment of albuterol with Atrovent mixed. While the patient is receiving his treatment, you establish an IV of normal saline and have given an initial bolus of 250 ml followed by a maintenance infusion of 500 ml/hr. While in route to the hospital, you decide to give a sq. injection of **.25 mg** of **Brethine** (terbutaline). On hand is a **1 cc** ampule containing **1 mg** of **terbutaline.** How many cc's will you give?

26. "Spring cleaning" is back in season. You have been dispatched to a woman having a **seizure.** When you arrive, you find a 36-year-old female lying in the front yard in a **postictal** state but **breathing.** The husband states that his wife was cleaning with **ammonia** and failed to open the windows. When he went into the house, he found his wife **coughing, vomiting,** and complaining about her **eyes burning.** As he got her outside, she started to seize, and that's when he called EMS. While your partner is securing the airway and giving oxygen, you establish an IV. As you finish taking the vital signs, which are **stable,** your patient begins to actively seize. According to protocol, you must administer **5 mg** of **diazepam** IVP. On hand is a **2 cc** prefilled syringe containing **10 mg.** How many cc's will you give?

27. It's **3:00 a.m.** in the middle of **January,** and you have been called out to an **infant** in **cardiac arrest.** When you arrive, you find the father performing **CPR** on his **4-month-old son.** While you are initiating aggressive ACLS protocols, the mother is telling you a little about her son's medical history. This **17**-year-old **mother** states that her baby was **premature,** weighing 4 pounds, but now weighs almost 9 pounds. She states that the only significant illnesses that he has had lately are a few **upper respiratory infections.** Upon contact with the baby, you note that the skin appears **mottled,** and you also notice **frothy, blood-tinged vomitus** in the baby's mouth. Even though you suspect that this infant is most likely suffering from **SIDS,** you must still continue to assure both the parents that everything possible is being done. When you hook up your Life Pak 5 monitor, you find that your patient is in **asytstole.** After initiating an intraosseous access, you must now administer **.01 mg/kg** of **epinephrine 1:10,000** IV. You recall that your patient's weight is **9** pounds. On hand is a **10 cc** prefilled syringe containing **1 mg.** How many cc's will you administer?

28. A call comes in for a man down in a warehouse. When you arrive, bystanders have a large fan blowing cool air on a man slumped against a wall. You quickly determine that your patient is in cardiac arrest. You do a quick look with defibrillator paddles and see fine **V-fib.** After vigorously following the V-fib protocol, your patient converts to **sinus bradycardia** with a palpable pulse of **30.** You administer **.5 mg** of atropine, and the HR increases to **50.** A few minutes have passed, and the patient's BP is **72/48.** According to protocol, it is necessary that you initiate a **dopamine drip** to be infused at **5 μg/kg/min.** On hand is a 10 cc vial containing **400 mg** of

dopamine, a **500 cc** bag of normal saline, and a **60 gtt** set. What would be the infusion rate with an estimated patient weight of **220** pounds?

29. EMS dispatch has received a call from Mac's Feed Store for a 45-year-old male experiencing **severe chest pain.** When you arrive, a bystander runs up to the ambulance and tells you to hurry. This bystander also advises you that **CPR** was started about 2 or 3 minutes ago. After establishing that **no pulse** was present, a quick look with the paddles reveals V-fib. You have performed your initial shocks, intubation, establishd an IV access, and given your initial dose of Epi. A few minutes into the code and after giving Cordarone, the patient converts into **torsades de pointes.** According to protocol, you must now give **2 gm** of **magnesium sulfate.** On hand is a **5 gm** vial in **10 ml.** With a patient weight of 300 pounds, how many ml's must you draw?

30. You have been dispatched to the residence of a 32-year-old female in **labor.** When the call came in, the husband advised that the infant was **crowning** and that this was her **fifth** child. Because this residence is about 40 minutes away, you are anticipating the mother will have already given birth when you arrive. Upon arrival, you find the infant in good health with an **apgar score** of **9.** While your partner is rendering care to the neonate, you proceed to evaluate the mother. The first thing you notice are the **blood-soaked sheets,** the delivery of the **placenta,** and the mother's **skin** color. You immediately instruct the husband to perform **fundal massage** while you attend to other treatment. Vital signs are P–**180,** BP–**90/60,** R–**36** and shallow; the skin is **pale** and **cool,** and you estimate that your patient has lost more than **500 cc** of **blood.** After giving oxygen, establishing two IVs of lactated ringers followed by a fluid bolus, and applying a perineal pad, you decide to immediately administer **10 units** of Pitocin. On hand is a **1 cc** tubex containing **10 units** of **Pitocin.** How many cc's must you give?

31. While standing by at the horse races, a spectator approaches and tells you that a man has **passed out** over by the barbecue booth. When you arrive, you find your patient to be in **cardiac arrest.** You promptly initiate **ACLS protocol.** Your patient is intubated, has an IV established, and has first-line drugs onboard. You're en route to the hospital and 15 minutes into the code. You are unable to convert your patient out of V-fib with the use of counter shocks, Epi, and amiodarone. According to protocol, your next drug of choice for V-fib is **Lidocaine.** You estimate your patient's weight at **145** pounds. You wish to give **1.5 mg/kg** of **Lidocaine** IVP. On hand is a **5 cc** prefilled syringe containing **100 mg** of **Lidocaine.** How many cc's will you push?

32. You have just been dispatched on a possible heart attack. Upon arrival, you find a 60-year-old male complaining of **chest pain.** The patient is **conscious** and **alert x 3,** and **diaphoretic.** The vital signs are BP–**140/100,** P–**120,** with respirations of **28.** The cardiac monitor is showing **sinus tachycardia.** You have administered oxygen and have established an IV access. You have been unable to relieve the patient's chest pain with Aspirin and sublingual nitro, so according to protocol you may administer **2 mg** of **morphine sulfate** IV. On hand, you have a **1 ml** vial containing **10 mg.** How many ml's will you draw?

33. Finally, you arrive back at the station after running back-to-back calls in the heat of the day. Just as the air conditioning starts to soak in, you receive a call to a rural residence with a response time of about 45 minutes. As you walk into this unbearably **hot** residence, you find a 54-year-old female in **respiratory distress** experiencing an **exacerbation** of her chronic emphysema. She advises you that she is a nonsmoker and that the only other history she has is CHF. After you give her four albuterol breathing treatments, she begins complaining of **nausea** and has a HR of **126.** Medical Control then orders you to initiate an **aminophylline infusion.** After you give her a loading dose, your order is to give **.5 mg/kg/hr.** The patient weighs **120** pounds. On hand is a **250 cc** bag of IV solution, **two** vials containing **250 mg** in each, and a **60 gtt** administration set. How many gtt/min must you administer?

34. While relaxing at the station watching the last 15 minutes of your favorite TV series, a car pulls up and someone knocks on the door. This person states that his mother's BP machine isn't working properly and asks you to check her BP. The patient is a 72-year-old female complaining of a **severe headache, visual disturbances,** and mild **anxiety.** When you check her BP, it is **260/150.** Suddenly, the patient begins to **vomit** and becomes **confused.** After securing a saline lock and giving oxygen, you decide to give **20 mg** of **labetalol,** slow IVP. On hand is a **20 ml** vial containing **100** mg of **labetalol** (Normodyne/Trandate). How many ml's must you draw to deliver the desired dosage.

35. You have received a call for an **asthmatic attack.** When you arrive, you find an extremely impatient 35-year-old female suffering from **status asthmaticus.** She stated that she was on her second Proventil treatment with no relief. Upon further evaluation, your patient is **cool** and **clammy,** with O2 sat of **94,** BP of **130/80,** P of **112,** R of **36** and **labored,** and **diminished** breath sounds. Your patient is **past** the **wheezing point** and progressing to where intubation may become necessary. You proceed to give three additional Proventil treatments with no relief. According to protocol, you must administer **.25 mg** SQ of **Brethine.** On hand is a **1 cc** ampule containing **1 mg** of Brethine. How many cc's must you draw to deliver the desired dose?

36. At 6:00 a.m. you receive a call for a medical emergency. When you arrive, you find an 80-year-old female who was awakened by her excruciating **chest pain.** Upon further evaluation, you find her to be **diaphoretic** with a BP of **88/42,** pulse of **100,** and respirations **36** and labored. The patient states that she has a cardiac history. After giving oxygen and aspirin, you hook the monitor up to find a sinus rhythm with bigeminy **PVCs** as well as short runs of **V-tach.** The patient states that she weighs about **150** pounds. Normally you would give this type of patient 1–1.5 mg/kg of **Lidocaine.** Because your patient is **over 70 years** of age, protocol states that you must give **half** the normal dose. You decide to give **.5 mg/kg** of **Lidocaine** IV. On hand is a **5 cc** prefilled syringe containing **100 mg** of **Lidocaine.** How many cc's must you give?

37. You have just received your paramedic certification, and you conclude that a good way to get your "feet wet" in the clinical field would be to get a part-time job at the hospital. Some days you'll be working in the ED, on other days you'll be assisting in the OB department. It is your second day on the job and you're working in the OB department. While taking a routine BP on a 27-year-old, you discover she is **hypertensive.** When you start to ask her how she feels, she begins to **shake.** Since the nurse had to run down to the ED, you immediately get on the phone and call her back. Two minutes later, as the nurse walks in, your patient starts to **seize.** She tells you to draw up **1 gm** of **magnesium sulfate.** On hand, you have a **20 cc** multidose vial containing **10 gm.** How many cc's must you draw?

38. Every now and then it becomes necessary to transport patients to Hilltop General Hospital, which is an hour away. You're en route with your 36-year-old patient who is receiving a blood transfusion. You have been on the road for about 15 minutes when you notice that your patient is experiencing **chills** and **flushing** of the **skin.** You check his vital signs, which reveal a BP of **82/64,** pulse of **150,** and respirations of **36** and labored. You immediately **stop** the blood transfusion and replace it with normal saline, because you feel your patient is experiencing a **transfusion reaction.** As you are contacting medical control, your patient becomes **unconscious.** Medical Control orders you to administer **50 mg** of **Benadryl** IVP. On hand is a **1 cc** vial containing **50 mg.** How many cc's must you draw to deliver the desired dose?

39. While you are assisting in the emergency department, a 54-year-old male is brought in by wheelchair and is complaining of **shortness of breath** and of a **severe headache.** On evaluation, you notice that the patient is extremely **diaphoretic.** His BP is **240/140** and respirations are **36.** The EKG monitor is showing sinus tachycardia with a HR of **112.** The ED doctor orders you to initiate a **Nipride drip** to run at **3 μg/kg/min.** On hand is a **50 mg** vial, a **250 ml** bag of IV solution, and **60 gtt** set. Your

patient states that he weighs **276** pounds. How many drops per minute must you deliver?

40. The county rodeo commission has requested that you stand by at the rodeo arena. A cowboy has just been thrown from the bull, and he isn't moving. You run into the middle of the arena "with a thousand people watching your every move" to find your patient **conscious** and complaining of **severe pain** in his left **shoulder.** He tells you that it is **dislocated** again, and sure enough, after further evaluation, you definitely agree with him. In an attempt to provide some pain relief, you need to administer **25 mg** of **Demerol** IM. On hand is a **1 ml** vial containing **50 mg.** How much do you need to draw from the vial to deliver the desired dose to this 165-pound patient?

41. Dispatch has just received an emergency call. When you arrive on scene, you find a 25-year-old female holding a blood-soaked rag on her foot. She is in **severe pain.** The patient states that she was mowing her yard with a push mower. She had no shoes on, and somehow her foot got caught under the mower. On exam, you see that **three** of her **toes** have been completely **amputated.** While your partner is outside looking for the **amputated** parts, you properly bandage the wounds. Your patient's vital signs are stable, and you have initiated an IV of lactated ringers. Since your ambulance does not carry any analgesics other than Nubain, protocol states that you may give **10 mg** of **Nubain** IV. On hand is a **2 cc** vial containing **20 mg.** How many cc's will you give?

42. While sitting around at the station watching the evening news, you're paged out on a sick call. When you arrive on scene, you find a 71-year-old male complaining of **dizziness** and of feeling **light-headed.** When you inquire about his medical history, he states that he has a history of rapid heart rate. His vital signs are BP–**100/P,** P–**180,** and R–**24.** When you apply the cardiac monitor, you discover that your patient is in **PSVT.** After attempting vagal maneuvers with no response, according to protocol, you

must administer 6 mg of adenosine rapid IVP. After giving the initial dose, your patient's condition is **unchanged.** You must now administer **12 mg** of **adenosine** rapid IVP, remembering to follow that with a rapid saline flush. On hand is a **4 cc** prefilled syringe containing **12 mg.** How many cc's must you administer in order to deliver the desired dose?

43. While working in the emergency department as an ER technician, EMS brings in a cardiac patient who has suffered an **MI.** Because the physician is involved in suturing a severe laceration with major bleeding, he instructs you to prepare a **heparin drip** while TPA is being prepared by the nurse. The physician's order is that you give a **loading dose of 5000 units** IV followed by **25,000 units** run over a **24-hour** time frame via drip. On hand, you have a **5 cc** vial containing **50,000 units** of heparin, a **1-liter** bag of normal saline, and a **minidrip** administration set.
    a. How many cc's would you draw for the loading dose?

    b. How many gtt/min would you deliver for the drip?

44. You've been dispatched on a pediatric emergency for a child shaking out of control. When you arrive, you discover a 15-month-old child in **status epilepticus.** The mother states that her child has had **coldlike symptoms** for the past few days and has been running a very high **fever.** While your partner is taking care of the airway and giving oxygen, you establish an IV of normal saline. You give .2 mg of Valium. It has now been a few minutes with no change in seizure activity. So, now you wish to administer .5 mg of **Valium.** On hand is a **2 ml** prefilled syringe containing **10 mg.** How many ml's must you administer?

45. New Year's Eve is starting off with a "bang." You've been called to the alley behind Mike's Bar & Grill for a possible **overdose.** When you arrive, your patient is still somewhat **responsive** but **combative.** Right away you notice that he is having **trouble** maintaining his **airway.** Your patient then begins to actively **seize.** After establishing a saline lock and after giving Valium, the patient is continuing to seize. His airway becomes of utmost importance and you have determined that this patient must be intubated as quickly as possible, but his **teeth** are **clenched.** It is then determined that a **neuromuscular blocking agent** is required in order to perform RSI (rapid sequence intubation). The patient's weight is estimated at **150** pounds. You've decided to administer **1 mg/kg** of **succinylcholine** (Anectine) IVP in order to relax the patient's muscles. On hand is a **10 cc** vial containing **200 mg.** How many cc's must you draw?

46. You have been dispatched to the Sunshine Day Care Center for a 6-month-old infant **not breathing.** Upon arrival, you find the care provider performing mouth-to-mouth. She describes the infant as being extremely **cyanotic** and that he had been in **respiratory arrest** for no longer than a minute or two when she began ventilations. Your patient is **unresponsive,** but a **pulse** is detected. However, the cardiac monitor shows sinus bradycardia with a HR of **80** and a BP of **70/54.** After securing the airway and **hyperventilating** the patient, you are unable to increase the infant's heart rate. Upon establishing an intraosseous access, you need to administer **.02 mg/kg** of **atropine** IV. You estimate the patient's weight at **15** pounds. On hand is a **10 cc** prefilled syringe containing **1 mg.** How many cc's must you give?

47. As soon as you walk into the station at 7:00 in the morning to begin your shift, you receive a call for a medical emergency. Upon arrival, the daughter of the patient meets you at the door. She states that her mother has **Parkinson's** disease and that she called her mother's neurologist after she called EMS. According to the daughter, her mother woke up this morning **nauseated,** and when she went to the bathroom, she became **weak** and **dizzy.** She also states that her mother can't seem to keep her **balance** and continuously keeps falling to her **left** side. While you are placing the patient on the stretcher, the neurologist calls the residence and requests to speak to the paramedic. After you relay a patient report to the physician, he states that it sounds like the patient

may be experiencing the beginning signs and symptoms of a **brainstem stroke.** He orders you to administer **8 mg** of **Decadron** IV. On hand is a **5 ml** vial containing **20 mg.** How many ml's will you draw?

48. You have been dispatched to a 68-year-old male complaining of **shortness of breath.** When you arrive, your patient states that he has emphysema and frequently feels his heart **skipping beats.** However, this time he tells you it is different because he is **light-headed** and feels like he can't **catch** his breath. While your partner is giving oxygen, you hook up the monitor to discover a sinus rhythm with multifocal **PVCs** and short runs of **V-tach.** After giving two doses of Lidocaine, bringing the total dose to 2 mg/kg of Lidocaine, the monitor is now showing occasional PVCs. You must now start a **Lidocaine drip** to be run at **3 mg/min.** On hand, you have a total of **two grams** of **Lidocaine,** a **500 cc** bag of normal saline, and a **60 gtt** administration set. At how many gtt/min must this drip be run?

49. You have been called to the residence of a 74-year-old female complaining of a **sudden** onset of **weakness.** Upon arrival, you find her to be **diaphoretic** with no chest pain. The daughter states that her mother has a history of high blood pressure and organic brain syndrome. When you take the patient's BP, you find that she is **hypotensive** with a BP of **60/42.** When you ask the daughter what medications her mother is on, she brings you a medicine bottle of labetalol tablets. When she hands it to you, she tells you that it was just filled yesterday and that it looks like **3** or **4** tablets are **missing.** The daughter then states that her mother's memory has gotten really **poor** and that it is highly possible that she may have taken some extra tablets. According to protocol, you must initiate a **dopamine drip** to be run at **4 μg/kg/min.** On hand is a 5 cc vial containing **200 mg,** a **250 ml** bag of normal saline, and a **minidrip** administration set. How many gtt/min must you deliver with a patient weight of **120** pounds?

50. You just put in your 8 hours at the office, and it's time to go home. Just 16 more hours of being on call, and it's vacation time. While you're eating dinner, the dispatcher pages you for a non-emergency transfer. This time you won't be transferring from the hospital to a residence in town. The patient's residence is 4 hours away. Your patient is being discharged following a post hip fracture. The patient is **stable,** and has **no** pertinent PMH. Two hours down the road, the patient begins to complain of **nausea.** Before you left the hospital, the doctor gave orders for Phenergan if the need arose. You have decided to give **25 mg** of **Phenergan** IM. On hand is a **2 cc** ampule containing **50 mg.** How many cc's must you give?

Answers

1. STEP 1   DD = **4 mg**

   STEP 2   C = 20 mg/5 ml = **4 mg/ml**

   STEP 3 $\dfrac{DD}{C} = \dfrac{4 \text{ mg}}{4 \text{ mg/ml}} = \textbf{1 ml}$

2. STEP 1   DD = **2 mg**

   STEP 2   C = 4 mg/10 cc = **.4 mg/cc**

   STEP 3 $\dfrac{DD}{C} = \dfrac{2 \text{ mg}}{.4 \text{ mg/cc}} = \textbf{5 cc}$

3. STEP 1   DD = **40 mg**

   STEP 2   C = 40 mg/4 ml = **10 mg/ml**

   STEP 3 $\dfrac{DD}{C} = \dfrac{40 \text{ mg}}{10 \text{ mg/ml}} = \textbf{4 ml}$

4. STEP 1   DD = **50 mg**

   STEP 2   C = 50 mg/2 cc = **25 mg/cc**

   STEP 3 $\dfrac{DD}{C} = \dfrac{50 \text{ mg}}{25 \text{ mg/cc}} = \textbf{2 cc}$

5. STEP 1   DD = **.5 gm**

    STEP 2   C = 1 gm/10 cc = **.1 gm/cc**

    STEP 3 $\dfrac{DD}{C} = \dfrac{.5\ \cancel{gm}}{.1\ \cancel{gm}/cc} = \textbf{5 cc}$

6. STEP 1   DD = .01 mg/kg $\longrightarrow$ $2.2\overline{)220}$ $\overset{10\,kg}{}$

                    $\longrightarrow$ 10 × .01 mg = **.1 mg**

    STEP 2   C = **1 mg/cc**

    STEP 3 $\dfrac{DD}{C} = \dfrac{.1\ \cancel{mg}}{1\ \cancel{mg}/cc} = \textbf{.1 cc}$

7. STEP 1   DD = **1 mg**

    STEP 2   C = 1 mg/10 cc = **.1 mg/cc**

    STEP 3 $\dfrac{DD}{C} = \dfrac{1\ \cancel{mg}}{.1\ \cancel{mg}/cc} = \textbf{10 cc}$

8. STEP 1   DD = 1 mg/kg $\longrightarrow$ $2.2\overline{)1400}$ $\overset{63.6\,\longrightarrow\,\textbf{64 kg}}{}$

                    $\longrightarrow$ 64 × 1 mg = **64 mg**

    STEP 2   C = 100 mg/5 ml = **20 mg/ml**

    STEP 3 $\dfrac{DD}{C} = \dfrac{64\ \cancel{mg}}{20\ \cancel{mg}/ml} = \textbf{3.2 ml}$

9. STEP 1   DD = 2.5 μg/kg/min $\longrightarrow$ $2.2\overline{)2000}$ $\overset{90.9\,\longrightarrow\,91\,kg}{}$

                    $\longrightarrow$ 91 × 2.5 μg = 228 μg

               DD = **228 μg/min**

    STEP 2   C = 250 mg/500 cc = .5 mg/cc

               $\longrightarrow$ .5 mg $\longrightarrow$ 500.μg = **500 μg/cc**

    STEP 3 $\dfrac{DD}{C} = \dfrac{228\ \cancel{\mu g}/min}{500\ \cancel{\mu g}/cc} = \textbf{.456 cc/min}$

    STEP 4 $\dfrac{cc \times gtt}{time} = \dfrac{.456\ cc \times 60\ gtt}{min} = 27.3 \longrightarrow \textbf{27 gtt/min}$

10. STEP 1   DD = 2 mg/kg $\longrightarrow$ $2.2\overline{)400}$ $\overset{18.1\,\longrightarrow\,18\,kg}{}$

                    $\longrightarrow$ 18 × 2 mg = **36 mg**

    STEP 2   C = **50 mg/cc**

    STEP 3 $\dfrac{DD}{C} = \dfrac{36\ \cancel{mg}}{50\ \cancel{mg}/cc} = \textbf{.72} \longrightarrow \textbf{.7 cc}$

11. STEP 1   DD = 1 mEq/kg $\longrightarrow$ $2.2\overline{)400}^{\,18.1}$ $\longrightarrow$ 18 kg

$\longrightarrow$ 18 × 1 mEq = **18 mEq**

STEP 2   C = 50 mEq/50 cc = **1 mEq/cc**

STEP 3 $\dfrac{DD}{C} = \dfrac{18\ \text{mEq}}{1\ \text{mEq/cc}} =$ **18 cc**

12. STEP 1   DD = **5 mg**

STEP 2   C = 10 mg/2 ml = **5 mg/ml**

STEP 3 $\dfrac{DD}{C} = \dfrac{5\ \text{mg}}{5\ \text{mg/ml}} =$ **1 ml**

13. STEP 1   DD = **.5 mg**

STEP 2   C = 1 mg/10 ml = **.1 mg/ml**

STEP 3 $\dfrac{DD}{C} = \dfrac{.5\ \text{mg}}{.1\ \text{mg/ml}} =$ **5 ml**

14. STEP 1   DD = **100 mg**

STEP 2   C = **100 mg/cc**

STEP 3 $\dfrac{DD}{C} = \dfrac{100\ \text{mg}}{100\ \text{mg/cc}} =$ **1 cc**

15. STEP 1   DD = 5 mcg/kg/min $\longrightarrow$ $2.2\overline{)2800}^{\,127.2}$ $\longrightarrow$ 127 kg

$\longrightarrow$ 127 × 5 mcg = 635 mcg

DD = **635 mcg/min**

STEP 2   C = 400 mg/250 cc = 1.6 mg/cc

$\longrightarrow$ 1.6 mg $\longrightarrow$ 1600.mcg = **1600 mcg/cc**

STEP 3 $\dfrac{DD}{C} = \dfrac{635\ \text{mcg/min}}{1600\ \text{mcg/cc}} =$ **.396 cc/min**

STEP 4 $\dfrac{cc \times gtt}{time} = \dfrac{.396\ cc \times 60\ gtt}{min} = 23.7 \longrightarrow$ **24 gtt/min**

16. STEP 1   DD = **.2 mg**

STEP 2   C = 1 mg/10 cc = **.1 mg/cc**

STEP 3 $\dfrac{DD}{C} = \dfrac{.2\ \text{mg}}{.1\ \text{mg/cc}} =$ 2 cc

17. STEP 1   DD = **10 mg**

STEP 2   C = 20 mg/2 cc = **10 mg/cc**

STEP 3 $\dfrac{DD}{C} = \dfrac{10\ \text{mg}}{10\ \text{mg/cc}} =$ **1 cc**

18. STEP 1   DD = **1 gm**

STEP 2   C = 5 gm/10 cc = **.5 gm/cc**

STEP 3 $\dfrac{DD}{C} = \dfrac{1 \text{ gm}}{.5 \text{ gm/cc}} = $ **2 cc**

19.   STEP 1   DD = 6 μg/kg/min $\longrightarrow$ $2.2\overline{)2000}$ $\dfrac{90.9}{}$ $\longrightarrow$ 91 kg

$\longrightarrow$ 91 × 6 μg = 546 μg

DD = 546 μg/min

STEP 2   C = 400 mg/250 cc = 1.6 mg/cc
$\longrightarrow$ 1.6 mg $\longrightarrow$ 1 6 0 0.μg = **1600 μg/cc**

STEP 3 $\dfrac{DD}{C} = \dfrac{546 \text{ μg/min}}{1600 \text{ μg/cc}} = $ **.341 cc/min**

STEP 4 $\dfrac{cc \times gtt}{time} = \dfrac{.341 \text{ cc} \times 60 \text{ gtt}}{\text{min}} = 20.46 \longrightarrow$ **21 gtt/min**

20.   **a.** STEP 1   DD = 30 mg/kg $\longrightarrow$ $2.2\overline{)1320}$ $\dfrac{60 \text{ kg}}{}$

$\longrightarrow$ 60 × 30 mg = **1800 mg**

STEP 2   C = 2000 mg/5 cc = **400 mg/cc**

STEP 3 $\dfrac{DD}{C} = \dfrac{1800 \text{ mg}}{400 \text{ mg/cc}} = $ **4.5 cc**

b. STEP 1   DD = **1800 mg/15 min**

STEP 2   C = 1800 mg/50 cc = **36 mg/cc**

STEP 3 $\dfrac{DD}{C} = \dfrac{1800 \text{ mg/15 min}}{36 \text{ mg/cc}} = $ **50 cc/15 min**

STEP 4 $\dfrac{cc \times gtt}{time} = \dfrac{50 \text{ cc} \times 60 \text{ gtt}}{15 \text{ min}} \longrightarrow \dfrac{3000 \text{ gtt}}{15 \text{ min}} = $ **200 gtt/min**

In reference to the answer for question 20**b**, after mixing the desired dosage into the 50 cc bag, the order was to run the bag over a time frame of 15 minutes. So, in essence, the only step that needed to be calculated was step 4, on calculating the drip rate.

21.   STEP 1   DD = **2 mg**

STEP 2   C = 10 mg/2 ml = **5 mg/ml**

STEP 3 $\dfrac{DD}{C} = \dfrac{2 \text{ mg}}{5 \text{ mg/ml}} = $ **.4 ml**

22.   STEP 1   DD = .05 mg/kg $\longrightarrow$ $2.2\overline{)380}$ $\dfrac{17.2}{}$ $\longrightarrow$ 17 kg

$\longrightarrow$ 17 × .05 mg = **.85 mg**

STEP 2   C = 8 mg/20 ml = **.4 mg/ml**

STEP 3 $\dfrac{DD}{C} = \dfrac{.85 \text{ mg}}{.4 \text{ mg/ml}} = \textbf{2.1 ml}$

23. STEP 1 $DD = 2 \ \mu g/kg/min \longrightarrow 2.2\overline{)1800}^{\ 81.8} \longrightarrow 82 \text{ kg}$

$$\longrightarrow 82 \times 2 \ \mu g = 164 \ \mu g$$

$$DD = \textbf{164 } \boldsymbol{\mu} \textbf{g/min}$$

STEP 2 $C = 200 \text{ mg}/250 \text{ cc} = .8 \text{ mg/cc}$

$$\longrightarrow .8 \text{ mg} \longrightarrow 8\underset{1}{0}\underset{2}{0}\underset{3}{0}. \mu g = \textbf{800 } \boldsymbol{\mu}\textbf{g/cc}$$

STEP 3 $\dfrac{DD}{C} = \dfrac{164 \ \mu g/min}{800 \ \mu g/cc} = \textbf{.205 cc/min}$

STEP 4 $\dfrac{cc \times gtt}{min} = \dfrac{.205 \text{ cc} \times 60 \text{ gtt}}{min} = 12.3 \longrightarrow \textbf{12 gtt/min}$

24. STEP 1 $DD = \textbf{4 mg/min}$

STEP 2 $C = 1 \text{ gm}/250 \text{ cc} \longrightarrow 1\underset{1}{0}\underset{2}{0}\underset{3}{0} \text{ mg}/250 \text{ cc} = \textbf{4 mg/cc}$

STEP 3 $\dfrac{DD}{C} = \dfrac{4 \text{ mg/min}}{4 \text{ mg/cc}} = \textbf{1 cc/min}$

STEP 4 $\dfrac{cc \times gtt}{time} = \dfrac{1 \text{ cc} \times 60 \text{ gtt}}{min} = \textbf{60 gtt/min}$

25. STEP 1 $DD = \textbf{.25 mg}$

STEP 2 $C = \textbf{1 mg/cc}$

STEP 3 $\dfrac{DD}{C} = \dfrac{.25 \text{ mg}}{1 \text{ mg/cc}} = \textbf{.25 cc}$

26. STEP 1 $DD = \textbf{5 mg}$

STEP 2 $C = 10 \text{ mg}/2 \text{ cc} = \textbf{5 mg/cc}$

STEP 3 $\dfrac{DD}{C} = \dfrac{5 \text{ mg}}{5 \text{ mg/cc}} = \textbf{1 cc}$

27. STEP 1 $DD = .01 \text{ mg/kg} \longrightarrow 2.2\overline{)90}^{\ 4 \text{ kg}}$

$$\longrightarrow 4 \times .01 \text{ mg} = \textbf{.04 mg}$$

STEP 2 $C = 1 \text{ mg}/10 \text{ cc} = \textbf{.1 mg/cc}$

STEP 3 $\dfrac{DD}{C} = \dfrac{.04 \text{ mg}}{.1 \text{ mg/cc}} = \textbf{.4 cc}$

28. STEP 1 $DD = 5 \ \mu g/kg/min \longrightarrow 2.2\overline{)2200}^{\ 100 \text{ kg}}$

$$\longrightarrow 100 \times 5 \ \mu g = 500 \ \mu g$$

$$DD = \textbf{500 } \boldsymbol{\mu}\textbf{g/min}$$

STEP 2 $C = 400 \text{ mg}/500 \text{ cc} = .8 \text{ mg/cc}$

$$\longrightarrow .8 \text{ mg} \longrightarrow 8\underset{1}{0}\underset{2}{0}\underset{3}{0} \mu g = \textbf{800 } \boldsymbol{\mu}\textbf{g/cc}$$

STEP 3 $\dfrac{DD}{C} = \dfrac{500 \cancel{\mu g}/min}{800 \cancel{\mu g}/cc} = .625\ \textbf{cc/min}$

STEP 4 $\dfrac{cc \times gtt}{time} = \dfrac{.625\ cc \times 60\ gtt}{min} = 37.5 \longrightarrow \textbf{38 gtt/min}$

29. STEP 1 DD = **2 gm**

STEP 2 C = 5 gm/10 ml = **.5 gm/ml**

STEP 3 $\dfrac{DD}{C} = \dfrac{2\ \cancel{gm}}{.5\ \cancel{gm}/ml} = \textbf{4 ml}$

30. STEP 1 DD = **10 units**

STEP 2 C = **10 units/cc**

STEP 3 $\dfrac{DD}{C} = \dfrac{10\ \cancel{units}}{10\ \cancel{units}/cc} = \textbf{1 cc}$

31. STEP 1 DD = 1.5 mg/kg $\longrightarrow$ $2.2 \overline{)1450}$ $\begin{array}{c} 65.9 \longrightarrow 66\ kg \end{array}$

$\longrightarrow 66 \times 1.5\ mg = \textbf{99 mg}$

STEP 2 C = 100 mg/5 cc = **20 mg/cc**

STEP 3 $\dfrac{DD}{C} = \dfrac{99\ \cancel{mg}}{20\ \cancel{mg}/cc} = 4.9 \longrightarrow \textbf{5 cc}$

32. STEP 1 DD = **2 mg**

STEP 2 C = **10 mg/ml**

STEP 3 $\dfrac{DD}{C} = \dfrac{2\ \cancel{mg}}{10\ \cancel{mg}/ml} = \textbf{.2 ml}$

33. STEP 1 DD = .5 mg/kg/hr $\longrightarrow$ $2.2 \overline{)1200}$ $\begin{array}{c} 54.5 \longrightarrow 55\ kg \end{array}$

$\longrightarrow 55 \times .5\ mg = 27.5 \longrightarrow 28\ mg$

DD = 28 mg/hr

STEP 2 C = 500 mg/250 cc = **2 mg/cc**

STEP 3 $\dfrac{DD}{C} = \dfrac{28\ \cancel{mg}/hr}{2\ \cancel{mg}/cc} = \textbf{14 cc/hr}$

STEP 4 $\dfrac{cc \times gtt}{time} = \dfrac{14\ cc \times \cancel{60}\ gtt}{(1\ hr)\ \cancel{60}\ min} = \textbf{14 gtt/min}$

34. STEP 1 DD = **20 mg**

STEP 2 C = 100 mg/20 ml = **5 mg/ml**

STEP 3 $\dfrac{DD}{C} = \dfrac{20\ \cancel{mg}}{5\ \cancel{mg}/ml} = \textbf{4 ml}$

35. STEP 1   DD = **.25 mg**

      STEP 2   C = **1 mg/cc**

      STEP 3 $\dfrac{DD}{C} = \dfrac{.25 \text{ mg}}{1 \text{ mg/cc}} = $ **.25 cc**

36. STEP 1   DD = .5 mg/kg $\longrightarrow$ $2.2\overline{)1500}$ $\dfrac{68.1}{}$ $\longrightarrow$ 68 kg

                   $\longrightarrow$ 68 × .5 mg = **34 mg**

      STEP 2   C = 100 mg/5 cc = **20 mg/cc**

      STEP 3 $\dfrac{DD}{C} = \dfrac{34 \text{ mg}}{20 \text{ mg/cc}} = $ **1.7 cc**

37. STEP 1   DD = **1 gm**

      STEP 2   C = 10 gm/20 cc = **.5 gm/cc**

      STEP 3 $\dfrac{DD}{C} = \dfrac{1 \text{ gm}}{.5 \text{ gm/cc}} = $ **2 cc**

38. STEP 1   DD = **50 mg**

      STEP 2   C = **50 mg/cc**

      STEP 3 $\dfrac{DD}{C} = \dfrac{50 \text{ mg}}{50 \text{ mg/cc}} = $ **1 cc**

39. STEP 1   DD = 3 µg/kg/min $\longrightarrow$ $2.2\overline{)2760}$ $\dfrac{125.45}{}$ $\longrightarrow$ 126 kg

                   $\longrightarrow$ 126 × 3 µg = 378 µg

                DD = **378 µg/min**

      STEP 2   C = 50 mg/250 ml = .2 mg/ml

               $\longrightarrow$ .2 mg $\longrightarrow$ 2 0 0 µg = **200 µg/ml**

      STEP 3 $\dfrac{DD}{C} = \dfrac{378 \text{ µg/min}}{200 \text{ µg/ml}} = $ **1.89 ml/min**

      STEP 4 $\dfrac{\text{cc} \times \text{gtt}}{\text{time}} = \dfrac{1.89 \text{ ml} \times 60 \text{ gtt}}{\text{min}} = 113.4 \longrightarrow$ **113 gtt/min**

40. STEP 1   DD = **25 mg**

      STEP 2   C = **50 mg/ml**

      STEP 3 $\dfrac{DD}{C} = \dfrac{25 \text{ mg}}{50 \text{ mg/ml}} = $ **.5 ml**

41. STEP 1   DD = **10 mg**

      STEP 2   C = 20 mg/2 cc = **10 mg/cc**

      STEP 3 $\dfrac{DD}{C} = \dfrac{10 \text{ mg}}{10 \text{ mg/cc}} = $ **1 cc**

42. STEP 1 DD = **12 mg**

STEP 2 C = 12 mg/4 cc = **3 mg/cc**

STEP 3 $\dfrac{DD}{C} = \dfrac{12 \text{ mg}}{3 \text{ mg/cc}} = \textbf{4 cc}$

43. **a.** STEP 1 DD = **5000 units**

STEP 2 C = 50,000 units/5 cc = **10,000 units/cc**

STEP 3 $\dfrac{DD}{C} = \dfrac{5000 \text{ units}}{10,000 \text{ units/cc}} = \textbf{.5 cc}$

b. STEP 1 DD = **25,000 units/24 hr**

STEP 2 C = 25,000 units/1 L
$\longrightarrow$ 25,000 units/1 $\underset{1\ 2\ 3}{0\ 0\ 0}$ ml = **25 units/ml**

STEP 3 $\dfrac{DD}{C} = \dfrac{25,000 \text{ units/24 hr}}{25 \text{ units/ml}} = \textbf{1000 ml/24 hr}$

STEP 4 $\dfrac{\text{cc} \times \text{gtt}}{\text{time}} = \dfrac{1000 \text{ ml} \times 60 \text{ gtt}}{24 \text{ hr}} \longrightarrow \dfrac{1000 \text{ ml} \times 60 \text{ gtt}}{1440 \text{ min}}$
$= 41.6 \longrightarrow \textbf{42 gtt/min}$

In reference to the above examples for question 43**b**, after mixing the desired dosage of 25,000 units into the 1-liter bag, the order was to run the **liter** over a time frame of 24 hours. So, in essence, the only step that needed to be calculated was step 4, on calculating the drip rate.

44. STEP 1 DD = **.5 mg**

STEP 2 C = 10 mg/2 ml = **5 mg/ml**

STEP 3 $\dfrac{DD}{C} = \dfrac{.5 \text{ mg}}{5 \text{ mg/ml}} = \textbf{.1 ml}$

45. STEP 1 DD = 1 mg/kg $\longrightarrow$ $2.2 \overline{)1500}$ $\overset{68.1 \longrightarrow 68 \text{ kg}}{}$
$\longrightarrow 68 \times 1 \text{ mg} = \textbf{68 mg}$

STEP 2 C = 200 mg/10 cc = **20 mg/cc**

STEP 3 $\dfrac{DD}{C} = \dfrac{68 \text{ mg}}{20 \text{ mg/cc}} = \textbf{3.4 cc}$

46. STEP 1 DD = .02 mg/kg $\longrightarrow$ $2.2 \overline{)150}$ $\overset{6.8 \longrightarrow 7 \text{ kg}}{}$
$\longrightarrow 7 \times .02 \text{ mg} = \textbf{.14 mg}$

STEP 2 C = 1 mg/10 cc = **.1 mg/cc**

STEP 3 $\dfrac{DD}{C} = \dfrac{.14 \text{ mg}}{.1 \text{ mg/cc}} = \textbf{1.4 cc}$

47. STEP 1 DD = **8 mg**

STEP 2 $C = 20 \text{ mg}/5 \text{ ml} = \textbf{4 mg/ml}$

STEP 3 $\dfrac{DD}{C} = \dfrac{8 \text{ mg}}{4 \text{ mg/ml}} = \textbf{2 ml}$

48.   STEP 1 $DD = \textbf{3 mg/min}$

STEP 2 $C = 2 \text{ gm}/500 \text{ cc} \longrightarrow 2\underset{1\ 2\ 3}{0\,0\,0} \text{ mg}/500 \text{ cc} = \textbf{4 mg/cc}$

STEP 3 $\dfrac{DD}{C} = \dfrac{3 \text{ mg/min}}{4 \text{ mg/cc}} = \textbf{.75 cc/min}$

STEP 4 $\dfrac{cc \times gtt}{time} = \dfrac{.75 \text{ cc} \times 60 \text{ gtt}}{min} = \textbf{45 gtt/min}$

49.   STEP 1 $DD = 4 \,\mu g/kg/min \longrightarrow 2.2\,\underset{1}{)}\overline{1200}\begin{array}{c}54.\textbf{5} \longrightarrow 55 \text{ kg}\end{array}$

$\longrightarrow 55 \times 4 \,\mu g = 220 \,\mu g$

DD = 220 μg/min

STEP 2 $C = 200 \text{ mg}/250 \text{ ml} = .8 \text{ mg/ml}$

$\longrightarrow .8 \text{ mg} \longrightarrow \underset{1\ 2\ 3}{8\,0\,0}.\mu g = \textbf{800 μg/ml}$

STEP 3 $\dfrac{DD}{C} = \dfrac{220 \,\mu g/min}{800 \,\mu g/ml} = \textbf{.275 ml/min}$

STEP 4 $\dfrac{cc \times gtt}{time} = \dfrac{.275 \text{ ml} \times 60 \text{ gtt}}{min} = 16.\textbf{5} \longrightarrow \textbf{17 gtt/min}$

50.   STEP 1 $DD = \textbf{25 mg}$

STEP 2 $C = 50 \text{ mg}/2 \text{ cc} = \textbf{25 mg/cc}$

STEP 3 $\dfrac{DD}{C} = \dfrac{25 \text{ mg}}{25 \text{ mg/cc}} = \textbf{1 cc}$

Index

Drip (*continued*)
  Nipride, 65, 88
  procainamide, 65
  rate calculation of, 59–63
Drop/drops (gtt), 60
Drug
  mixing of, 59–63

E
Epinephrine, 28, 32, 45, 73, 77, 83

F
Flumazenil, 78

G
Glucagon, 43
Gram (gm)
  conversion to milligram (mg), 2

H
Haldol, 72
Heparin drip, 89

I
Injections, 49–53
Insecticides, 80–81
Intramuscular (IM) injection, 49–53
Intraosseous (IO) injection, 49–53
Intravenous (IV) injection, 49–53
IV drip, 40

K
Kilogram (kg)
  pound (lb) conversion to, 3–5

L
Labetalol, 86
Lasix, 40, 42, 51, 72
Lidocaine, 30–32, 51, 55, 59, 64, 66, 74, 81,
    85, 87, 91
Liter (L)
  conversion to milliliter (ml), 2–3

M
Macrodrips, 60
Magnesium sulfate, 79, 84, 87
Microgram (μg)
  milligram (mg) conversion to, 2
Midazolam, 80
Milligram (mg)
  conversion to microgram (μg), 2
  gram (gm) conversion to, 2

Milliliter (ml)
  liter (L) conversion to, 2–3
Minidrip, 60, 75
Morphine sulfate, 85

N
Naloxone, 45
Narcan, 28, 72
Nipride drip, 65, 88
Nubain, 89

O
Organophosphate poisoning, 81
Overdose
  cocaine, 76
  tricyclic, 76
  Valium, 78

P
Per (/), 27
Phenergan, 92
Pitocin, 84
Pound (lb)
  conversion to kilogram (kg), 3–5
Procainamide, 63, 65

R
Romazicon, 78

S
Sodium bicarbonate, 30, 76
Solumedrol, 79
Stadol, 44
Subcutaneous (sq) injection, 49–53
Succinylcholine, 90

T
Terbutaline, 82
Thiamine, 77
Time factor, 52
Tricyclic overdose, 76

U
μg. See microgram

V
Valium, 31, 43, 50, 76, 90
  overdose, 78

W
Whole numbers, 3, 4, 5